CHAMPIONSHIP NUTRITION AND PERFORMANCE:

The Wrestler's Guide to Lifestyle, Diet and Healthy Weight Control

Nicholas Rizzo, M.D.
Team Physician and Wrestling Coach

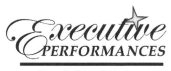

Executive PERFORMANCES

Publishing

an imprint of
Executive Performances, Inc.

CHAMPIONSHIP NUTRITION AND PERFORMANCE:
The Wrestler's Guide to Lifestyle, Diet and Healthy Weight Control

© 2003 by Nicholas Rizzo. First Edition: October, 2003. Revised Edition: January, 2004. All rights reserved.

Executive Performances Publishing, an imprint of Executive Performances, Inc.
P.O. Box 93, Palos Park, Illinois, 60464
www.executiveperformances.com

ISBN: 0-9748220-1-9 (Comb bound)

ISBN: 0-9748220-0-0 (Paperback)

Library of Congress Control Number: 2003116611

This book is printed on acid free paper.

Printed in the United States of America

The information contained in this book, including opinions and recommendations, is intended to provide a broad understanding and knowledge of nutrition and health topics as they specifically relate to the sport of amateur wrestling, and is for educational purposes only. It should not be considered complete and is not intended to be a substitute for medical, psychiatric, or psychological evaluation and treatment. No one should act upon any information provided in this book without first seeking medical advice from a qualified medical physician. Always consult your physician before beginning any exercise or diet program. Individual nutritional needs and results will vary.

There is little scientific data available regarding diet and nutrition in pre-adolescent athletes. Consequently, it may not be necessary or advisable for pre-adolescent athletes to follow a strict diet/nutrition regimen, aside from following a healthy diet in general. The composition, amounts and timing of meals for teenage athletes must be carefully supervised.

Notify your parents, coaches and physician immediately if you don't feel well, if you have any questions or problems, or if you have any medical problems requiring special or individualized dietary or athletic needs. For help with any physical problems, weight problems, or emotional problems associated with eating problems or eating disorders, talk to your physician and a mental health professional.

Any activity involving motion, height, wall collisions or physical contact creates the possibility of serious injury, serious injury, which may include permanent paralysis or even death. Wrestling mats do not totally eliminate this hazard. Wrestling, training or competition should be done under the supervision of trained and qualified coaches and instructors at all times. Know your limitations and follow progressive training practices. Be sure to consult your coaches and instructors. Inspect mats prior to any activity. Specifically identify any deterioration of the covering and/or foam material of the mat. Ensure the integrity of mats mounted to wall surfaces. Repair or replace as required. Mats are often constructed in sections. These sections may move during the use of the mat. Check for proper fastening (taping) prior to use. Mat protection will vary according to room temperature. For wrestling purposes, always follow current National Collegiate Athletic Association (NCAA), National Federation of State High School Association (NFSHS), or International Federation of Associated Wrestling Style (FILA) Standards and Guidelines.

CONTENTS

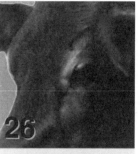

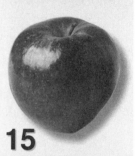

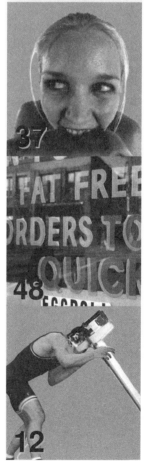

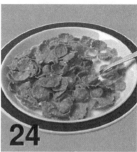

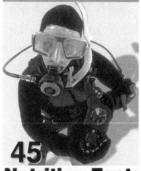

WRESTLING HANDOUT #1: Cauliflower Ear
WRESTLING HANDOUT #2: Concussions
WRESTLING HANDOUT #3: Head Injury Fact Sheet
WRESTLING HANDOUT #4: Guidelines for Parents of
  Children in Sports
WRESTLING HANDOUT #5: Herpes & Cold Sores
WRESTLING HANDOUT #6: Hygiene & Health
WRESTLING HANDOUT #7: Illness Prevention
WRESTLING HANDOUT #8: Impetigo
WRESTLING HANDOUT #9: Muscle Cramps
WRESTLING HANDOUT #10: Nosebleeds
WRESTLING HANDOUT #11: Ringworm & Tinea
WRESTLING HANDOUT #12: Rules of the Room
WRESTLING HANDOUT #13: Skin Care
WRESTLING HANDOUT #14: Strains & Sprains
WRESTLING HANDOUT #15: When to Use Heat &
  Cold for Athletic Injuries

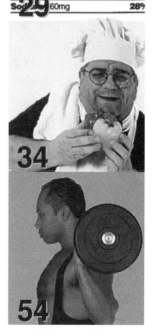

ACKNOWLEDGEMENTS

Endless thanks go to my brother, Mark Rizzo, who has always been an inspiration, and a source of knowledge and support, both in the sport of wrestling and in life; and to my parents Judy and Nick for suffering through hours upon hours of "bleacher butt". Special thanks are extended to Mark Gervais, who is not only an exceptional coach and mentor, but also a friend. My gratitude is extended to Lynn Miner, Ph.D., Brian Farrell, M.D., Lela Iliopoulos, R.D., L.D., Brad Janecek, Mike Quirk, Amanda McCann, and Patricia Pierson for their review and attention to this book. Sincere thanks also go to Al Ferreira, Don Kotara, Jack Griffin, Alan Fried, and Pat Quirk. I'd like to extend appreciation to J.R. Harris and Jill Weimer for their help answering my 1001 questions about publishing. Finally, Becky Pate, Shanda Henderson, and Kevin Clark at Central Plains Book Manufacturing in Winfield, Kansas also deserve thanks for helping make this book a reality.

Nicholas Rizzo, M.D.
January 2004

PREFACE FROM "THE WRESTLER'S DIET"[1]

A very well-done educational brochure entitled "The Wrestler's Diet" was written in 1991 by Roger Landry, M.A., Robert Oppliger, Ph.D., Ann Shetler, R.D., L.D. and Gregory Landry, M.D., made possible by a grant from The Quaker Oats Company. It has since been placed on the Internet in various forms. The excellent Preface by Roger Landry from "The Wrestler's Diet" says it all, and is presented here.

"In high school, I wrestled varsity at 98 pounds my freshman year and at 105 pounds as a sophomore. I didn't have to cut weight either year. In my junior year, I weighed 140 pounds before the start of the season. Although I was determined to wrestle varsity again, I couldn't beat any of the number one wrestlers within 20 pounds of my weight. I thought my only alternative was to drop to 112 pounds. I decided to go for it. My days of care free weight control were over."

"I had no idea how much fat I had to lose, and I didn't care. I made up my mind that I was going to make 112 pounds no matter what. When I started my diet, I didn't eat anything for the first two days and then limited my food intake to about 700 calories per day. I worked out in rubber suits and sat in saunas to lose fluid weight. I drank very little water or other liquids. I made weight at 112 pounds and won my first match. I was feeling healthy and strong and was convinced that I had done the right thing. I celebrated by pigging out at a fast food restaurant. I was nine pounds overweight the next day."

"Throughout the season, I ran, starved, sweat, and spit before each match in order to make weight. After each weigh-in, I rewarded myself by eating, usually in excess, before I wrestled. I repeated this cycle every match. Gradually, my performance began to suffer. My strength was progressively decreasing, and I was always tired. I started losing matches I should have won. It was difficult to concentrate in classes, and my grades started to slip. I was always hungry. Losing weight before each match became increasingly more difficult. I even resorted to using laxatives. My desire to wrestle was becoming overshadowed by my desire to eat. I was constantly thirsty. My skin was dry, itchy, and cracking from dehydration. I was miserable. I quit the team before the end of the season. I played basketball my senior year."

"It wasn't until I became a wrestling coach that I regretted what I had done that season. I realized cutting so much weight made me hate a sport I truly loved. If I had applied myself as much to my wrestling as I had to making weight, I might have been a much better wrestler."

"As a coach, I am determined to prevent my wrestlers from making the same mistakes. I want them to concentrate on their wrestling and not on their weight so they can enjoy the sport of wrestling. It is the coach's responsibility to teach wrestlers the right information on nutrition and weight control. The Wrestler's Diet was developed specifically for wrestlers and their parents, but is also intended to help wrestling coaches teach the principles of proper nutrition."

Roger Landry, Wrestling Coach

INTRODUCTION - HOW TO USE THIS BOOK

Wrestling is fun, exciting, builds character and teaches self-knowledge. Unfortunately, improper methods of weight loss and poor nutrition take away from those benefits. All too often, wrestlers believe that to be a better wrestler they must lose a lot of weight to move down one or more weight classes, or that punishing themselves by losing more weight makes them tougher. These are simply not true. Wrestlers do best when managing their weight properly through nutrition and correct training, and competing at their proper weight.

Also, like many young athletes, wrestlers often eat whatever is available and often forget that proper nutrition is an important part of gaining that competetive edge. Wrestlers often have the unhealthy idea that all food is "fat-producing". They forget that food provides energy and vital nutrients to fuel and build their bodies. Think of your body like a car. If you put cheap gas in your car, it will run poorly. If you do not put any gas in your car (like starving your body) it will not run at all. Similarly, imagine putting fuel in your body to make your muscles run. Good nutrition is about knowing what foods and fluids make your muscles run best. It is about fueling your body at the right times and in the right amounts with the right types of food that will boost your daily energy, performance and health.

Wrestlers who do not practice proper nutrition end up doing unhealthy or inappropriate methods of weight loss and cannot perform at their best. Inappropriate weight loss occurs from dehydration, improper nutrition, improper training, or eating disorders and includes:

- ✓ Too much weight loss
- ✓ Too rapid weight loss
- ✓ Cycling of weight (repeated rapid loss and gain)

When wrestlers become dehydrated or fast too much their performance suffers and it takes about five hours for initial physical recovery, and up to two to three days for full recovery. New wrestling rules have moved weigh-ins up to one to two hours prior to competition in an effort to keep wrestlers from dehydrating and fasting too much. Wrestlers should emphasize year-round conditioning and nutrition to maintain a steady healthy weight, instead of doing unhealthy weight practices to lose weight quickly near to and during the wrestling season.

More importantly, unlike most athletes who tend to earn better grades during sports seasons, wrestlers are likely to experience poor focus and concentration, mood swings and tiredness resulting in lower grades during the wrestling season. Some of these problems appear to be from low blood sugar (hypoglycemia) from fasting as well as by the many bad effects of dehydration. One study showed decreased short-term memory in college wrestlers who "cut" too much weight, and who did it in the wrong way. Also, wrestlers should not rely on diet alone to manage their weight. (See "How Conditioning and Weight Training Relate to Weight Control" on page 13.)

Like many other sports, what is really important is not your weight but your body make up. Using the "fat-lean" model of body composition the combined weight of fat mass and lean mass equals total body weight.[13] Because weight alone does not discriminate between fat and muscle, it is a poor measure of body composition. Weight gain is either desirable or undesirable depending on whether fat or muscle is increasing. The best situation is to have an increase in muscle (lean mass with an increase in strength) with a maintenance or lowering of fat (extra weight). So weight itself is a poor predictor of success, *but fitness is.*

This book was written to help wrestlers get the full benefits of the sport by achieving their peak performance as close to their minimum natural weight as possible without compromising their health. This book is not about "cutting weight", but instead about getting the right calories and nutrients from the right sources, knowing how conditioning and training apply to this, and avoiding lifestyle mistakes that can hurt you. Also, it's intended to help wrestlers learn life-long, healthy eating habits that will benefit them long after they have stopped competing. As it makes a big difference if coaches and parents take an active role in meal planning and make sure that a variety of healthy foods are easily accessible, this book is written for wrestlers on all levels, coaches, trainers and parents.

The chapters in this book apply to different degrees to different age groups and levels of wrestling, but it is recommended that you read this book in its entirety. For example, wrestlers under 10 years of age should not focus on weight control, so chapters like "Weight Certification" are not as relevant to them. As significant growth occurs in the high school years, chapters like "Weight Class Certification" are very important to high school wrestlers. As you go up on your level of competition, chapters like "Nutrition" and how it relates to weight control *and* performance increase in importance. So some chapters are more relevant to college wrestlers than grammar or high school wrestlers. But chapters like "Eating Before Competition" and "Dehydration" are important for *all* levels. Important "take home messages" are printed in bold or italics, or are placed in boxes like the one below.

- ♦ **Focusing on becoming a better wrestler instead of focusing on losing weight will make you a better wrestler.**

- ♦ **To grow naturally and increase strength wrestlers need the same nutrients as other people but need more calories and hydration to meet the demands of daily training.**

- ♦ **Losing weight gradually (1.5% of your total weight per week – about 1 pound for a 103 pound wrestler, 2 pounds for a 150 pound wrestler, and 3 for a heavyweight) is the best way to lose fat and keep muscle.**

- ♦ **Achieving peak physical and mental performance requires proper nutrition every day. This includes the day *of* and *after* competition.**

- ♦ **Losing weight rapidly (inappropriate weight loss), poor nutrition, fasting, and dehydration may limit growth, decrease strength and power, increase body stress, decrease the ability to think clearly, and increase risk of injury and illness. *These effects cannot be completely reversed in the time between weigh-in and competition.***

THE PARENTS' ROLE IN A YOUNG WRESTLER'S HEALTH*

The age of the wrestler plays a big role in how closely one should manage their weight. In general, beginner's wrestling can occur as early as four or five years of age, but true competition should wait until wrestlers are at least seven or eight years old. Many kids do not really enjoy competition until age ten or 11. To gain overall development and an appreciation of sports in general, kids should not specialize in a single sport until they are in high school or college. In most cases, children over ten years of age can begin serious training for wrestling.[8]

> **Concern with weight management should not begin until a wrestler is at least ten years or older.**

The parents' goal here should be overall health for the young athlete. From a dietary standpoint, do the following: [29]

- ◆ Control the food, not the children. Buy healthy food and have it easily accessible. Don't react positively or negatively to a child's eating preferences – this will lead to an aversion to the food later on in life. One particularly bad thing parents can do is to buy junk food, and then punish a child for going for it.

- ◆ Keep offering rejected foods. Getting kids to develop preferences for healthy foods isn't always easy. Wait a few days to two weeks and re-offer a rejected food. Typically, they will accept it anywhere between the second and fifteenth time, depending on their age.

- ◆ Be sure your child is getting enough calories and proper nutrients like calcium in their diet.

- ◆ Limit juice and soft drinks. Too much juice or soda is associated with childhood obesity. Try to opt for water or low-fat milk. If you must have soda, then choose diet soda.

- ◆ Set a good example. Kids are very in-tune to parental preferences. For example, children of picky eaters are more likely to be picky eaters themselves.

- ◆ Sit down to a family meal. At a family meal the food is more likely to be healthy, kids are more likely to eat it, and they are less likely to eat junk food and soft drinks throughout the day.

- ◆ Turn off the TV. Studies have shown that children eat bad food and more of it in front of the television. Limit television to one and a half hours a night.

- ◆ Avoid fast food. Studies show that kids that eat fast food eat more food more often and are more obese.

*Refer also to WRESTLING HANDOUT #4: Guidelines for Parents of Children in Sports

WHAT DETERMINES YOUR "NATURAL" WEIGHT?

"I'm not overweight. I'm just nine inches too short."
– Shelley Winters

Several things determine a person's natural height and weight. Growing taller is determined by genetics and nutrition, with height and bone strength mainly determined by age five. An adequate amount of calories and good nutrition are critical to ensuring that growth and energy demands are met in order for a young athlete to grow to his/her full potential. Aside from getting enough calories and nutrition to maintain growth, there is nothing a person can or should do to "get taller" or "bigger". Factors affecting how fat or skinny a person is include genetics, activity level, diet and eating patterns, age and metabolism (how fast your body burns calories). Things affecting metabolic rate include age, gender, body composition, growth rate, medications, and nutritional state. Fat regulating hormones may also be a factor.

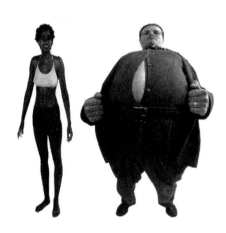

Eating patterns are the amount you eat, how and when you eat, and any healthy or unhealthy eating patterns. Psychological factors may also play a role in someone's weight in healthy or unhealthy ways ("emotional eating" is one example). Psychological problems here may also include eating problems related to stress or depression, or eating disorders like anorexia or bulimia.

Another factor is the age – an obese child may slim down during adolescence, a thin adolescent may gain additional muscle and/or fat as his/her frame grows, or the opposites may even happen. Hormones (like testosterone) and their changing levels play roles here also.

When you take in fewer calories, your body "downshifts" its metabolism. This leads to a return to your original weight because you are expending less energy. In other words, the less you eat, the less you can eat to maintain weight. It also makes sense that a 20% increase in calorie intake will lead to a 20% increase in weight. However, although weight gain does occur, it does not increase as much as you would expect – your body adjusts its energy output again. However, when you overfeed to gain weight, the amount of weight gain is proportionate to the amount of overfeeding. This suggests that we have a fat "set point" or "fat thermostat" (homeostatic mechanisms) that helps keep us at our "natural" weight during times of changing caloric intake. This is probably a survival mechanism of our bodies that helps us survive periods of famine and store energy as fat during times when extra food is available. The way to override this mechanism is by gradually changing your lifestyle by eating healthier and establishing exercise regimens that increase your metabolism.

It is important to realize that every person's body composition is different and your goal should be to maintain a healthy weight and fitness level appropriate for your age, build and current level of training and activity.

DETERMINING YOUR WRESTLING WEIGHT

"People tell me not to lose weight – I might lose my personality. I tell them, 'Honey, my personality ain't in my thighs.'"
– Oprah Winfrey

The goal here is to achieve your "in-shape weight" or "minimum wrestling weight" for competition. At your "in-shape weight" you will have speed, agility, strength and focus. Your proper weight class should not be so low that you have to sacrifice your health or performance in order to make weight. In addition to the bad physical effects, unhealthy weight loss practices affect you mentally; the more you worry about your weight the less you can concentrate on your wrestling.

What's your fightin' weight?

BOTTOM LINE: Not everyone needs to lose weight. You, your parents and coaches should all be informed on what proper weight management is. And all should help decide your proper weight class (while not going below your certified minimum weight). *This should be based on your performance on the mat, in school and at home.* If any of those areas suffer, something is wrong and you need to find out what it is – trying to lose too much weight, being out of shape, poor nutrition or hydration, not managing stress well, too much pressure from parents or peers, or anything else.

Weight alone is a poor indicator of your fitness, and a poor indicator of how much success you will have. If you find yourself focusing only on weight, consider the following: unlike body weight (where changes are frequently seen on a daily basis due to things like hormone shifts and hydration) real changes in body composition (from less fat to more muscle) take time. And they show up first in places other than on a scale. Muscle weighs more than fat, so the scale will not reflect this healthy change at the beginning. Because muscle is heavier than fat, the changes you may notice are that you feel stronger and more energetic and that your clothes fit looser. Yet neither of these changes is shown on a scale – a scale cannot tell between fat and muscle. Pay attention to the other changes and decrease the emphasis on the scale. Keep the big picture in mind.

Some wrestlers will end up on an emotional roller coaster because of what the scale says they weigh. If your mood is determined by your weight, you need to change your perspective. Do not let the scale dictate how you feel. There is much more to this sport than what you weigh. So you must keep your short and long-term goals in mind.

> **Most importantly, pay attention to your energy level and how you feel during workouts and throughout the day. This is the best way to see if you are managing your weight, diet and lifestyle correctly.**

Weight Class Certification

Many states now require wrestlers to be certified at a minimun wrestling weight class that they are then not allowed to compete below. The main points are best expressed in this excerpt from "Weight Management – Changing a Culture", by Sam Crosby, Chair, NFHS Wrestling Rules Committee, written in 2001.

> Over the last several years, the NFHS Wrestling Rules Committee has adopted rules that attempt to discourage wrestlers from losing extreme amounts of weight. The most significant rules include:
>
> ◆　Requiring each wrestler to establish a certified minimum weight before January 15.
>
> ◆　Prohibiting a wrestler from wrestling more than one weight class above the certified weight without recertifying at a higher weight.
>
> ◆　Recommending body fat measurements and hydration levels in establishing a minimum certified weight.
>
> ◆　Prohibiting the use of sweatboxes, vinyl suits, diuretics or other artificial means of quick weight reduction.
>
> ◆　Permitting wrestlers to have a two-pound growth allowance.
>
> ◆　Requiring shoulder-to-shoulder weigh-ins one hour before the start of a dual meet and two hours before tournaments.
>
> This year, the rules committee made a strong statement in revising the weigh-in procedure – a statement that emphasizes the importance of safety in urging wrestlers to wrestle as close to their natural weight as possible. With the new weigh-in rules, wrestlers may not leave the weigh-in area once they report to weigh in; nor may they engage in any activities in the weigh-in area that encourage dehydration. In dual-meet competition, wrestlers at weigh-in may step on and off the scales only three times, to allow for possible discrepancies in scales, and in tournaments, the wrestlers may step on each available scale one time to make weight. With the new weigh-in procedures, it is hoped that everyone connected with wrestling will begin to move away from an emphasis on the sport of cutting weight to concentrating on the sport of wrestling.

Most states have now adopted these or similar weight certification rules – *as different states may have different rules, be sure to check with your state as to their specific guidelines.* The NWCA (National Wrestling Coaches Association) has created an excellent Weight Certification Internet Calculator Program, available at www.nwcaonline.com. You must be a member of the NWCA to use this program. The NWCA calculator requires skinfold or underwater weighing measurements, and other information about each wrestler.

The NWCA program's benefits and goals include:

1. Determining a lowest allowable weight class for each wrestler
2. Establishing a safe weight loss/weight gain plan
3. Producing all necessary compliance forms
4. Delivering the program to the scholastic and collegiate community for nominal cost
5. Providing an opportunity for wrestlers to build a customized diet that honors their weight loss/weight gain plan

Percent Body Fat and Measurement Methods[2, 13, 16]

The term "body composition" generally refers to how much muscle and fat you have. "Lean weight" refers to the weight of your body's functioning tissues: muscles, bones, kidneys, heart, skin, etc. "Fat weight" is how much your fat weighs. "Body fat percentage" is the percent of your body made up of fat. Your minimum wrestling weight can easily be determined through body fat percentage measurements (a measure of your body composition). But keep in mind that these numbers are not necessarily your ultimate goal. Your goal is to get into a range of weight, and not to an arbitrary fat percentage.

The purposes of determining your body composition though body fat percentage measurements include:

♦ Finding out where your body composition is now, both to get a "starting point" and to identify any problems associated having with too much or too little fat

♦ Determining your ideal body weight and minimum body weight (or weight class) in order to help you avoid improper weight loss it's problems

♦ Developing a plan and timeline for appropriate weight loss, if indicated

♦ Follow your progress throughout the course of the season

Scientific methods for measuring body fat percentage are not perfect, but are only estimates to use as guides. Since each method uses different ways of estimating body fat, cross-comparisons between methods should *not* be made. Because each method has different errors in the way they measure things, and different people have different errors in each method, it would be a mistake to compare two values from different methods to determine how your body has changed over time. For instance, if you had your body fat percentage measured using skinfolds last year and had a 4% error in the heavier direction, and you used bioelectrical impedance analysis (BIA) yesterday and had an error of 3% in the lighter direction, combining these would result in an error of several pounds.

Below are some of the methods of scientifically determining body fat percentage, with the two most commonly used methods being underwater weighing and skinfold measurements.

Underwater Weighing: This is also called "hydrostatic weighing". Overall, this and DEXA (Dual Energy X-ray Absorptiometry) are the gold standards, with underwater weight being the standard that other methods are typically compared to. While both underwater weighing and DEXA have high costs and limited availablity, hydrostatic weighing is more widely used as it is more available and less costly compared to DEXA.

Underwater weighing works on the idea that your weight under water is directly proportional to the volume of water displaced by your body (the "Archimedes Principle"). Because body fat makes you more buoyant, the difference between your in-water weight and out-of-water weight can tell you how much body fat you have. First, you are weighed on a standard scale to get a "land weight". Then, the volume of your lungs is estimated by blowing into a tube on a device that measures air volume. Next, you sit in a special weighing chair and exhale as much air as possible before being lowered under shoulder-high water for a few seconds and your underwater weight is read.

While there is some error related to your hydration status and the remaining air in your lungs, this method is quite good for determining the change in body fat percentage over time. Disadvantages of underwater weighing are that it requires special, bulky equipment and trained personnel to perform the tests. For some people, it is too uncomfortable to exhale completely and remain under water even for a few seconds. In such cases, another method like skinfolds or Bod Pod would be better.

Below are some tips that will make underwater weighing easier and more effective.

♦ Avoid heavy exercise for eight to 12 hours prior

♦ Avoid gassy foods for two days prior

♦ Fast for four hours before the test

♦ Be hydrated

♦ Practice breathing all the way out and then holding your breath a few times

♦ Bring a swim suit and take off any jewelry

Skinfold Measurements: One way that has become common due to it's accuracy, reliability and inexpensive cost is by measuring the thickness of certain skinfolds on the body. This method requires individuals to have their skin slightly pulled and pinched by the technician's hand and caliper. Skinfolds indirectly measure a double thickness of the fat layer under the skin (subcutaneous fat). This fat layer represents about half of a person's total body fat. The results of the skinfold measurements will give you a good estimate of your total body fat level. For example, if the results indicate a body fat reading of 14%, that simply means that 14% of your body is fat. Such measurements are only estimates, and the error is about ± 2% to ± 9% for skinfold testing, depending on the user and the specific calculations used. In this example, you could be 12% to 16% fat (14% ± 2%). Skinfold measurements should be performed by healthcare professionals experienced with them. Things such as age, gender and other demographics can affect skinfold accuracy. Skinfold results can be very useful as relative values (whether you have lost, gained or stayed the same) when measured under similar conditions.

The calculations used with skinfolds are reasonably reliable as they are derived from underwater weighing results. However, you need to be sure that the body fat calculations being used are the right set of equations. There are different equations for different populations. Unfortunately, all too often the equations used with athletes are actually meant for the general population. Since many athletes are leaner than average people are, they end up with inaccurately low results when using calculations designed for the general population. So using the right calculations and equations specific to the population being measured gives results that are more accurate.

For the general population, calculations that use more skinfold measurements are generally more accurate. For example, one set of calculations may require height, weight, age, triceps skinfold and an abdomen skinfold. Another set of calculations may require height, weight, age, and skinfolds at the triceps, subscapular, midaxillary, suprailiac, abdomen and midthigh. As the errors in these different sets of calculations are different, it would be a mistake to compare one value with another that was obtained using a different set of skinfolds and a different equation. For wrestlers' bodies, it has been found that certain specific sites are consistent and accurate – the subscapular, abdominal, and triceps for males and the abdominal and triceps for females. These are the sites required for the NWCA Weight Certification Internet Calculator Program.

Keep in mind that skinfold measurements are more accurate when you are well-hydrated. Proper skinfold weight certification must include a urine test (called specific gravity) that measures your level of hydration. You will be asked to provide a sample of urine and it will be tested with a medical urine dipstick to see how much water is in the urine – a reflection of your level of hydration.

Tips for passing the specific gravity urine test include:

♦ Avoid foods that cause water loss like caffeine, soda and chocolate for 24 to 48 hours prior

♦ Avoid *all* types of supplements

♦ Avoid heavy exercise for 24 hours prior

♦ Avoid being tested in the early morning (when you are dehydrated from not drinking fluids during the night)

♦ Drink plenty of fluids for a few days before – see "Hydration Guidelines" on page 45

<u>DEXA Scanning</u>: DEXA stands for Dual Energy X-ray Absorptiometry and was originally developed to determine bone density in diseases like osteoporosis. It is the latest, most accurate, and most expensive way of determining body composition. It uses calculations and weak X-rays to estimate bone, fat and lean soft-tissue mass. Bacically, you lay on the DEXA table for about 20 minutes, the X-rays pass through your body, and the machine measures the amount of X-ray that has been absorbed by the different types of tissues it passed through. The higher the tissue density, the greater the decrease in X-ray intensity. (Do not worry about the X-rays' negligible effect on your body. The amount of X-ray used is extremely small. One regular chest X-ray has about 800 times the X-ray radiation of DEXA.)

<u>Bod Pod</u>: This is also called Plysmography or Air Displacement Plethysmography. It works on the same idea as underwater weighing except that is uses air instead of water. It requires the person to sit inside an oxygenated chamber for four minutes while the chamber uses air and pressure changes to calulate your body fat percentage. Advantages to this method are that it is highly repeatable and reliable, it's a bit faster and safer than underwater weighing, and it's not as vulnerable to human error. It's main disadvantage is that it is only available at certain locations like universities or hospitals.

<u>Bioimpedance</u>: BIA is a fast and relatively inexpensive method. It is a reliable technique, but the results are not as accurate as compared to underwater weighing. BIA requires you to be in contact with two electrodes applied to the hand, wrist, foot and/or ankle. A safe, low-level electrical signal is passed through your body, and the opposition to the flow of electricity (called impedance) is measured with the BIA analyzer. Water transmits electricity well (conducts), and most body water is in your lean mass. Fat is such a poor conductor of electricity that it actually slows (impedes) the flow of electricity. So it follows that the greater the impedance, the greater the level of fat. As the amount of water in your system affects how well the electricity conducts, it is important that you are hydrated when doing a BIA measurement. Drinking alcohol, exercising, drinking a lot of coffee, and spending a lot of time outside in hot weather within 24 hours of a BIA test will make the results less accurate. Consequently, you should do BIA after a day of rest and be sure that you are properly hydrated. Advantages to BIA are that it is fast, easy to use, noninvasive and it does not require specially-trained personnel. Drawbacks to BIA include it's expense and that it may not be as valid in younger athletes.

<u>Computerized Calipers</u>: These are like skinfold calipers but have built-in computers that do the body fat percentage calculations themselves. The drawbacks to these are, as with regular skinfolds measurements, they may or may not have the right calculations for young athletes and may be more expensive than standard skinfold calipers.

Minimum Body Fat

One of the main goals of safe weight loss is to *lose excess fat weight.* Not all fat on your body can be considered "excess" fat. A certain amount of fat is needed for use as energy, to act as a shock absorber for your internal organs, to insulate your body from the cold and to store certain nutrients.

Teenagers should not be doing excessive calorie restriction and they should not skip meals. The second biggest growth spurt occurs during adolescence. Limiting calories during these years could limit growth. For most teenage males, the normal range of body fat percentage is 7% to 20%, with 10% to 15% being ideal. For most teenage females, the acceptable body fat range is 12% to 25%, with a range of 15% to 20% considered ideal.[2] *When a person drops below these fat percentages, they may not be getting enough calories to support growth during the "growth spurt" years. These percentages are a bit lower for college wrestlers because most of their growth spurts have already occurred.* (See "Losing and Maintaining Weight" on page 12.)

While male college wrestlers sometimes achieve 5% body fat, 7% is generally considered the lowest healthy fat level for teenage males. Male wrestlers should not be competing in a weight class where their body fat percentage is below 7% if they are under 16 years of age, or below 5% if they are 16 or older. Female wrestlers should not be competing in a weight class where their body fat percentage is below 12% if they are under 16 years of age, or below 10% if they are 16 or older.

Wrestlers with lower body fat percentages cannot afford more weight loss without significant losses of muscle, strength and endurance. Keep in mind that 7% and 12% are not magic numbers — just guidelines to follow.

Because different wrestlers react differently both mentally and physically to dieting and dehydration, there is no one perfect fat percentage that applies to everyone. Most wrestlers perform very well at a higher percentage of body fat, especially the heavier weight classes. So, if you are now 10% body fat, there is no reason to believe that you'll wrestle better at 7%.

On occasion, because of genetics or ethnicity, some young athletes' natural weight may place them below the 7% minimum body fat for males and 12% minimum for females. A physician familiar with young athletes should be asked to verify that the wrestler is healthy and fit, and give written medical clearance that the athlete can safely participate at a particular weight. Before a physician medically clears a young athlete below 7% body fat (12% if female), a pattern of weight should be documented, and there should be no evidence of malnutrition, eating disorders or unhealthy levels or types of exercise.[2] In addition, most states' rules on weight certification will not allow a wrestler with less than 7% body fat (12% for females) to lose any more weight, nor compete at a weight class below what he/she weighs. Check with your state's specific guidelines.

This guy is way more than 7% fat!

LOSING AND MAINTAINING WEIGHT

"How long does getting thin take?"
  – Winnie the Pooh, <u>Winnie the Pooh</u> by A. A. Milne

Assess your body fat percentage and determine your minimum weight class before the season starts. Once you've determined your weight class, you should next develop a plan for getting to and staying at your target weight. Ideally, you should have most of your fat loss done by the start of the season. If you plan ahead, a gradual and responsible reduction in weight can be easily accomplished.

> **Try to stay fit and maintain healthy weight throughout the entire year. A healthy diet should be started in the summer so healthy eating patterns are established and can easily be followed during the wrestling season. Plan your diet to lose no more than 1.5% of your weight each week. For example, if you weigh 150 pounds and want to lose 10 pounds, allow *at least* 5 weeks (2 pounds per week) to reach your goal. Weigh yourself before and after practices to monitor your fluid weight loss but monitor your fat weight loss by weekly weight changes.**
>
> <u>**Remember:**</u> **Healthy weight loss requires eating a balanced diet that supplies enough calories to support growth and daily activities, and drinking enough fluid to maintain a good state of hydration.**

Also, do not mistake water loss for fat loss. For example, a 151 pound wrestler with a 14% body fat could get down to 135 pounds by reducing to 7% body fat and then undergo very little, if any dehydration. It would be foolish for the same wrestler to reduce to only 144 pounds (10% body fat) by dieting and then dehydrating 7 to 10% for a weigh-in and have his performance suffer. On the other hand, if a wrestler seems to be losing because he is getting outmuscled time and again, and if the fat percentage estimate indicates he has fat to lose, he may try a lower weight class. A wrestler should *never* be forced by coaches, parents or peers to go down to a lower weight class.[9]

One concern about weight loss for young wrestlers is the potential for hindering normal growth. Male teenage growth spurts typically occur between the ages of 12 and 16. *Restricting calories too much in order to reach an unrealistic weight during these years could hinder growth.* But there is little evidence that following a healthy diet with adequate intake of calories and nutrients has a negative effect on growth (see "Eating Disorders and Wrestlers" on page 56.)

HOW CONDITIONING AND WEIGHT TRAINING RELATE TO WEIGHT CONTROL

"An ounce of prevention is worth a pound of cure."
   – Henry de Bracton

Exercise and conditioning (and to some degree weight training) is the main factor in determining body composition. Don't rely on diet alone to lose weight.

Different types of exercise place different types of stresses on your body, and the body responds differently to each of these. Types of exercise can be generally categorized into two groups: aerobic (cardiovascular, typically low-intensity and longer duration like long-distance running) and anaerobic (typically high-intensity and of short duration like weight lifting). For the most part, any type of activity (aerobic or anaerobic) will reduce body fat. High-intensity activity may increase muscle and reduce body fat, so the decrease in weight may be minimal (you are trading fat weight for muscle weight). This kind of change in your body is likely to make you appear slightly smaller, because, while still weighing the same, lean muscle mass takes up less space than fat. In contrast, low-intensity activity appears to reduce body fat percentage while adding little muscle, so both body fat and weight are reduced. When exercising and burning the same amount of calories in aerobic or anaerobic activity, body fat is reduced to the same extent. One way to look at it is that while both

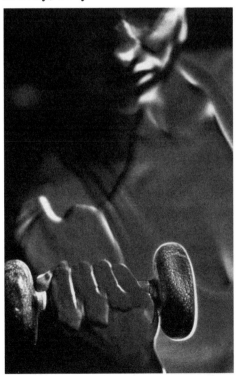

aerobic and anaerobic activity reduce your body fat, aerobic training improves your conditioning and raises your metabolism, while weight-training increases muscle mass. As a form of workout, wrestling lies somewhere in between these two types of activities. In other words, wrestling has both aerobic and anaerobic components. That is why the best wrestlers usually look more muscular than runners, and less muscular than professional body builders.

One important key to weight control and fitness is to combine both types of activities. After you work out aerobically, your metabolism (the rate at which your body burns calories) is raised for the next several hours, burning more calories the whole time. If you increase your muscle mass through strength training, the extra muscle you gain also burns calories at that higher metabolic rate during those several hours. So they work together to accomplish this (called synergy).

Strength is not developed or kept up by doing only wrestling. The old approach was to lift weights in the off-season to increase muscle size and strength with the hope that a wrestler could maintain or minimize losses in strength during the season by doing only wrestling and then fasting and deydrating to make weight. This was never a very good strategy to begin with, and with the new requirements for body-fat testing and hydration this will never work. Consequently, a weight program should be part of a your year-round routine. During the season, weight training helps to maintain muscle mass and strength by combating muscle loss during times of tightly controlled caloric intake. Studies have shown that some wrestlers may become weaker as the season goes on, so it's important to do strength training three to four times a week.

To have conditioning play it's proper role in weight control, follow your coaches' advice and:

- ◆ Use a year-round approach to maintaining an appropriate weight and body composition.

- ◆ Combine some aerobic activities with different types of strength training for variety. Activities that do this include running hills, sprints, circuit training, isometric exercises and speed drills. Only do exercises or drills that are cleared by your coach.

- ◆ Keep extra workouts outside of regular practices short (under 30 minutes) so your body can recover.

- ◆ Remember that good conditioning and proper weight training help prevent injuries.

- ◆ For safety reasons and for proper form, you must weight train with a partner.

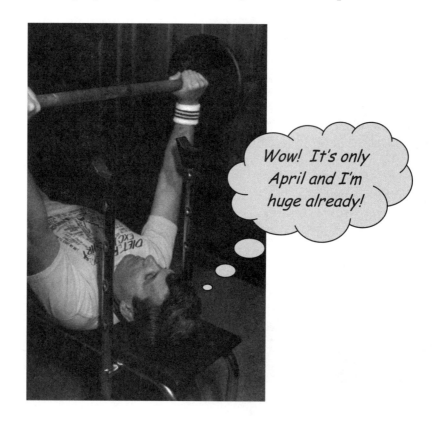

NUTRITION

A balanced diet plan that includes all the food groups will allow you to get all the nutrients in the amounts you need for your growth and training. To manage your diet the right way, you will need to understand things like proper diet, hydration, when to eat, and other things covered in the following chapters. The United States Department of Agriculture (USDA) Food Guide Pyramid is a healthy eating plan for people ages two and over. It shows the recommended number of servings to eat from each of five food groups every day to meet your nutrition needs, and it defines serving sizes.[25] Keep in mind that these recommendations are guidelines designed for people in general, and your individual requirements as an athlete may be different from this. If you are trying to control your weight and fitness, getting enough calories should be the main priority, while at the same time including the proper amounts of dietary components like fats, protein, carbs, vitamins, minerals and fluids. Some experts feel that an athlete's diet should differ from the general guidelines and should consist of 20% fats, 15% protein and 65% carbs. A general rule is to have ½ your plate filled with fruits and vegetables, ¼ with starchy foods like pasta or potatoes, and ¼ with protein like beans, meat, fish or poultry.

The USDA's Food Pyramid

The Food Pyramid guidelines give the *minimum* number of recommended servings from each food group for each day. The menus in Appendix B show some examples. The Pyramid is divided into four levels according to the needs of your body.

The bottom of the Pyramid contains foods like whole grains such as oats, rice and wheat, and the whole breads, cereals, noodles and pasta made from them. Six to 11 servings of these are recommended each day. These are high in carbohydrates, which are the main

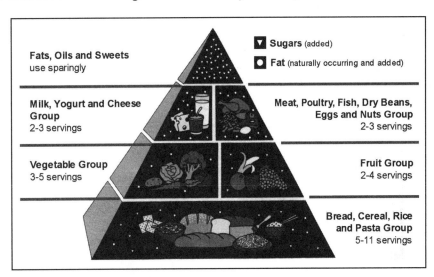

energy source for training and other body functions.

The second level includes foods from the vegetable and fruit groups. These include all fresh, frozen, canned and dried fruits and vegetables, and juice. These groups are loaded with vitamins, minerals, carbohydrates, water and fiber. Consequently, they can satisfy your hunger with fewer calories than other types of foods. Recommendations are to have ten servings of fruits and vegetables each day. Fruits contain a natural sugar called fructose, which will not cause a rapid rise in blood sugar like the one processed or added sugars will. So they are better for you. But you still need to be aware of portion sizes as fruit is moderately high in calories. Do not expect proper weight and fitness if you eat 30 cantaloupes a day!

The third level has two food groups: the dairy products including milk, yogurt and cheese; and the meat and meat alternative foods including meat, poultry, fish, dry beans, eggs and nuts. These groups are rich in proteins, vitamins and minerals, and are essential for healthy bones and muscles. Choose low-fat dairy products and lean (low-fat) meat products to get the full advantage of these foods without extra fat calories. Your diet should include two to three low-fat servings from the dairy group and two to three servings (six to nine ounces total) from the meat group each day.

The top level includes nutrients that should be used sparingly in your diet, including fats, oils and added sugars. Many of these are already present in foods already discussed and are often added in processed foods. Be careful in your choice of foods and check labels for added sugars and fats that can add calories to your diet without increasing their nutritional value. Choose unsaturated fats over unhealthy saturated fats. (See "Fats" on page 25.)

The "Athlete's Food Pyramid"

The USDA's Food Pyramid is a good guide for the general population. But there is debate about how it does or does not reflect more recent nutritional research, and an intensely-training athlete's needs may be different. Below is a proposed "Athlete's Food Pyramid". It includes the ideas of having the base of the pyramid for Fluids (as suggested by the Gatorade Sports Science Institute[®][24]), splitting up the carbs into "good" and "bad" carbs, and splitting the fats into "good" and "bad" fats as proposed by Dr. Walter C. Willett[28]. In addition, the minimum recommended servings for some categories have been increased to provide some (and only possibly needed) extra protein without additional bad fats, and additional good carbohydrates for energy during training and competition. Most importantly, you need to keep in mind that these are *suggested guidelines only*, and you need to meet your *individual* energy and fluid needs on a daily basis.

Use sparingly

Red Meat and Butter | Pasta, Sweets, Potatoes, White Rice, White Bread

Dairy Foods or Calcium Supplement
2 - 3 Servings

Fish, Poultry and Eggs
1 - 3 Servings

Nuts and Legumes
2 - 4 Servings

Vegetables (in abundance) | Fruits 4 - 5 Servings

Whole Grain Foods and Breads (at most meals) | Plant Oils (Olive, Canola, Soy, Corn, Sunflower, Peanut, and other vegetable oils)

Fluids
See "Water and Other Fluids" on page 20 and "Hydration Guidelines" on page 45

"Anywhere" Guide to Serving Sizes

These serving sizes are from the Food Guide Pyramid and are based on suggested and usual portions needed for good nutrition. *They are different than the serving sizes on the Nutrition Facts Label, which reflects portions typically eaten.* Below are some handy references for determining approximate serving sizes.

Visual Comparison	Approximate Measurement	Serving Example
Thumbnail	1 teaspoon	1 serving butter or oil
1 egg	1 ounce	1/3 serving lean meat
Thumb or 2 dominoes	2 ounces	1/2 serving cheese
Ping-pong ball	2 tablespoons	1 serving peanut butter
Palm of hand or a deck of cards	3 ounces	1 serving meat, poultry or fish
Scoop of ice cream	1/2 cup	1 serving dry beans or chopped vegetables
Fist, a large handful or a baseball	1 cup	1 serving dry cereal 1 serving leafy vegetable 2 servings pasta or potatoes

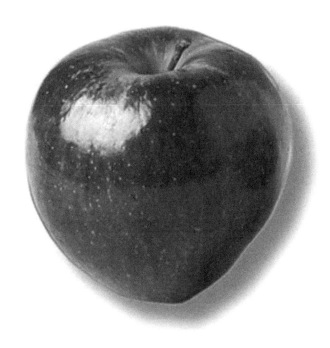

CALORIES

A calorie is a unit used to describe the energy content of foods. Energy is stored in your body as glycogen (stored in the muscles and liver) and as fat. When you take in more calories (energy) than you use, those extra calories are stored as fat and you gain weight. Weight loss occurs when you consume fewer calories than you use. Your body can break down fat, glycogen or muscle protein for energy. Which of these it uses depends on how much energy you need and how quickly you need it. Losing weight gradually causes your body to break down its stored fat for energy. Losing weight too rapidly causes your body to break down muscle proteins for energy.

In planning your diet it is helpful to estimate how many calories you need each day. Caloric needs differ from wrestler to wrestler depending on things like an individual's metabolism, fat percentage, body size and activity level. No two wrestlers are alike, and wrestlers in the same weight class may have different caloric needs. You can estimate the *minimum* number of calories you need each day by using the graph in Figure 1. Appendix B contains examples of 2,000 to 3,500 calorie menus to help you plan your diet. Keep in mind that if your workouts are sluggish, if you are tired during the rest of the day, or if you are fatiguing out as the season goes on you may not be eating enough calories or hydrating enough.

You must burn 3,500 calories to lose one pound of fat. You can lose one or two pounds of fat a week by burning 500 to 1,000 more calories a day than you take in. Burning more than that leads to loss of muscle.

> **Gradual weight loss is best accomplished by combining your training with a slight reduction in calorie intake. Your calorie intake should not fall below 2,000 to 3,000 calories per day (depending on your size and training and activity level). If you do extremely rigorous training, you should have at least an additional 1000 calories per day. <u>Most athletes require between 3,000 and 6,000 calories a day</u>.**

Figure 1.

Determine the <u>minimum</u> number of calories for your goal weight.

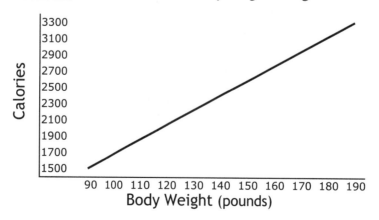

For example, if you are a high school wrestler and weigh 150 pounds, your minimum caloric intake should be 2500 calories, according to the graph in Figure 1. To make up the calories needed in workouts, add anywhere from 300 to 500 calories *per workout* depending on the type of workout and intensity level (a college wrestler should add up to 1000 calories for an intense wrestling practice). In this example, if you run or lift weights in the morning (200 to 300 calories) and then you have a typical wrestling practice in the afternoon (500 calories), you need to eat an extra 700 to 800 calories that day, and these should be made up with mostly carbs. So your daily caloric intake should be around 3300 calories. If you need to lose a few pounds (you should drop no more than 1.5% of your body weight per week), then take away about 500 calories, leaving 2800 calories a day (3300 for college wrestlers). One general guideline: get 500 extra calories for every hour of intense wrestling practice.

Keep in mind, your fat and protein intake should meet the requirements for your weight, and the extra calories adjusted by adding carbs according to your total caloric needs. You should calculate the calories you get from your protein and fat requirements based on your weight (see "Protein" on page 26 and "Fats" on page 25 for these guidelines and calculations). Then subtract this amount of calories from the your total required calories for the day. The difference between these should be made up with carbs.

For example, a 150-pound high school wrestler should be eating 67.5 grams of fat per day (0.45 grams of fat x 150 pounds). That equals 607.5 calories (67.5 fat grams x 9 calories per fat gram). He should also be eating a minimum of about 61 grams of protein a day (between 0.36 and 0.45 grams of protein x 150 pounds). As a typical American diet includes much more protein than we need, let's estimate this number at 100 grams of protein that he just happens to eat on a normal day. That would equal 400 calories. So the calories he eats from fat and protein approximate 1000. And if he is at his desired weight and needs to take in 3300 calories total, that would leave 2300 calories he should be getting from carbs.

Calorie Burning Calculator (Adapted from www.mrtrainer.com)

Below is a reference chart for calories burned for an average male, 5'10" and 175 pounds (80 kg). To convert these to *your* calories burned during an activity, locate on the chart which exercise you did and estimate to within the nearest 15 minutes how long you exercised. Place the number of calories burned for the average male (from the chart) into the following equation: (Your weight ÷ 175) x chart number = your total calories burned.

EXERCISE	15 min.	30 min.	45 min.	60 min.
Circuit Training (with weights)	185	320	455	580
Cycling (12 mph)	100	200	300	410
Football	140	280	390	530
Jumping Rope	170	290	460	620
Running (6 min mile pace)	280	555	815	1160
Running (10 min mile pace)	180	360	540	730
Stair Climber	155	310	460	618
Walking (17 min. mile pace)	65	130	200	275
Weight Training	130	270	385	510
Wrestling (5 min. matches)	225	450	700	965

NUTRIENTS AND OTHER DIET COMPONENTS

There are six essential groups of nutrients you need to build and fuel your body every day: water, carbohydrates, protein, fats, vitamins and minerals. To get energy from foods, it is important to know about what to eat and when. While your body needs nutrients from all six categories to perform well, three of them provide energy for training: protein, fats and carbs. After you eat, these three are released into your bloodstream and converted to blood sugar (glucose) – your body's main source of energy. Energy that is extra or not used right away is stored as glycogen or fat. Glycogen is glucose stored for quick release during times of exercise. Most glycogen is stored in your liver, with smaller amounts in your muscles. Consider fat as energy in long-term storage.

Water and Other Fluids

Water and fluids are often overlooked as an important part of good nutrition. A minimum of three to four quarts of fluids such as sports drinks, water, juices, decaffeinated beverages or milk should be a part of your daily diet. It is important to drink plenty of fluid during practice and between matches. Not only will you feel better, but you may also find you have more endurance and energy during practice and throughout the day.

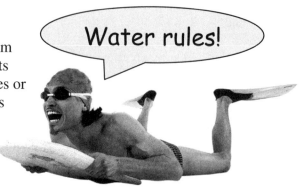

Water rules!

Water: Your body is 60 to 70% water. A fluid loss of 2 to 3% of your weight can quickly occur during intense training. *A wrestler may lose up to three to four quarts of water during an intense practice.* Drinking enough water is the single most important thing an athlete can do for good nutrition.

Milk: Milk is a good source of protein, vitamins and minerals. Drink reduced fat or skim milk instead of whole milk, as this will make a big difference in caloric and fat intake. An 8 oz. glass of skim milk has 0.4 grams of fat and 85 calories, 2% milk has 2.5 grams of fat and 120 calories, and whole milk has five grams of fat and 150 calories. Do not drink milk before competition if it upsets your stomach.

Juices: Natural fruit and vegetable juices are good during the day. They are a great source of vitamins and minerals, and are easily digested. The sugars in juices are natural sugars (like fructose and lactose) and are good for your body – not like the added, processed sugars in junk food. Some athletes drink juices diluted to 50% to 75% with water for quick "drinkability." If a juice has a lot of carbs (sugars) it should be diluted down to only 8% carbs if you drink it on competition days.

But there are some catches with natural juices. They lack sodium, and the fructose in them is absorbed more slowly than other forms of carbs (sugars), and so they are not ideal to hydrate with immediately before, during or immediately after workouts or competition.

Another drawback to juices is that drinking too much juice as a child has been associated with long-term obesity. But this has not been studied much in child athletes. In general, pre-teens should have no more than one to two glasses of juice a day and instead focus on water and low-fat milk. (One exception to this may be drinking juice as an after-workout snack.) For adult athletes, fruit juices are great and should be part of a daily diet and hydration plan. Be careful: not all juice is "juice." Be sure to check labels on vegetable and fruit drinks for additives like large amounts of sodium or excessive amounts of added sugars. (See "How to Read Food Labels" on page 29.)

Sports drinks: These are another great option for hydration, especially during competition and workouts. In this book the term "sports drinks" refer to the clear liquid drinks like Gatorade® and function as energy sources but also are fluid replacements. Properly formulated sports drinks (6% carbohydrate or 14 g/8 oz) are somewhat more quickly absorbed and effective at replacing fluids than water, soft drinks or juice. But there are three main types of nutritional supplements considered "sports drinks" and you should know their differences:

1. Sports Drinks (fluid replacements): These drinks are absorbed quickly and are great for hydration and some carb reloading during and after workouts and competition. Examples of these include Gatorade®, Max® and Powerade®. As hydration is a main point in wrestling, these types of drinks are great for wrestlers. Advantages of sports drinks include:

   ♦ They help delay fatigue by providing carbohydrates (energy) during exercise.

   ♦ Athletes have been shown to drink more of a flavored beverage than plain water and then hydrate a bit better.

   ♦ They help the body retain more fluid in the muscles.

   ♦ They provide electrolytes (like sodium and potassium).

   ♦ Unlike other fluids, they have the amounts of carbs and sodium that promote quick hydration and absorption – they help your body hang on to fluid.

2. Carb Loaders: These are often thick liquids or gels. They are high in carbs and reload muscle glycogen during or after workouts. They are often used by elite athletes during long endurance sports like marathons. These usually have carbs greater than 8% and are not recommended during exercise as hydrators, but rather as "energy sources". Examples of these include Gatorlode® and Carboplex®.

3. Nutritional Supplements (sports shakes): These are high in vitamins and minerals in addition to carbs. They are often used in place of a high fat meal during the week, or as an easily digestable meal during long tournament days. Examples of these include Gatorpro® and Exceed Sports®.

Beware of other additives in drinks labeled as "sports drinks". For example, some so-called "sports drinks" have herbal ingredients, caffeine or other additives, all of which can cause problems.

Soft drinks: Both regular and diet sodas should be avoided, especially during workouts. Disadvantages of soft drinks include:

♦ They consist of "empty calories" and provide nothing of value to the body.

♦ They may be associated with obesity in children.

♦ They are high in sugars and may cause a large insulin release resulting in increased hunger a little while later. Also, the sugar in most of these is fructose, which is not as quickly absorbed as other carbs.

♦ Carbonated beverages are less likely to help with hydration because they are ten to 11% carbs and are consequently slower absorbed. They may also reduce the amount of good fluids you can take in.

♦ The carbonation in soft drinks turns into carbon dioxide gas in your stomach and gut. When you drink soft drinks, especially quickly or in large quantities, they may cause bloating and stomach cramps.

♦ Many soft drinks contain large amounts of caffeine which can promote deyhydration and should be avoided (see "Caffeine" on page 62).

Beware of oversized drinks (24 ounces or more). Eight ounces of soda has about 140 calories – 24 ounces of pop would be 420 calories or nearly 20% of your daily calories in a 2,000 calorie diet. Also, if you are drinking too much soda, you may not be taking in enough healthy fluids. Focus instead on water or fluids that provide nutrients along with appropriate calories. Fruit juices, low-fat milk and sports drinks are much better choices.

> **Bottom Line**: Drink fluids like water, juices, lowfat milk and sports drinks throughout the day. Drink sports drinks and/or water before, during (about every 20 minutes) and after workouts.

Carbohydrates

Carbohydrates are the main fuel source for your muscles and brain and should provide most of your calories. Fat is used as an energy source during long, endurance types of work like marathons. Even wrestlers with low body fat percentages have fat available as a source of energy. Carbs, on the other hand, break down into sugar (glucose), which is then either used right away or stored as a type of carb called glycogen in the muscles and liver. Because carbs break down faster than fats, they are the main source of energy for high-intensity, maximal-outburst work like wrestling. One way to look at it is that while protein is used to build and repair muscles and fat is long-term energy storage, carbs *move* the muscles.

But stores of carbs are in short supply in your body. As many wrestlers typically do not eat enough carbs, its very important for them to keep up on their carbs. Most carb sources are easy to digest and are great snacks for wrestlers. Eating the right carbs at the right times maintains training intensity and helps with quick recovery.

In order to know which carbs to eat and when, you need to be familiar with the term "glycemic index" (how fast a carb breaks down and makes your blood sugar rise over the next few hours). A carb's glycemic index affects when and how fast energy is available to you, so paying attention to it makes sense. If a carb causes your blood sugar to rise more quickly than other carbs, then it has a high glycemic index. If it enters the bloodstream slowly, it has a low glycemic index. For example, foods with carbs "trapped" in lots of fiber release carbs more slowly (low glycemic index). How a food is prepared or eaten can also have an effect on a food's glycemic index. For example, eating the skin of a fruit or vegetable lowers the index as it often has most of the fiber.

With regard to wrestling, think of carbs in three groups: "Life", "Quick Energy", and "Garbage" carbs as follows.

Life Carbs: These "good" carbs are healthy carbs that you should be eating on regular days and on the days prior to competition. **"Life" carbs are very healthy, natural, are usually high-fiber, are not processed and have low to moderate glycemic indices.** (These good carbs are sometimes called "complex" carbs.) Fiber slows glucose absorption so you do not get a rapid rise in blood sugar, which causes a big insulin release with more hunger later. These high-fiber carbs have another benefit: they increase the bulk of the meal, making you feel fuller before you get too many calories (see "Fiber" on page 24). This helps you regulate how much you eat. Try to get most of your carbs from "good" carb sources. But keep in mind that high-fiber good carbs, while they are more nutritious than refined carbs, have just as many calories. If a low-glycemic index carb is digestible, you can eat it prior to exercise. Most fruits are good carbs. But some release their energy quicker than others. High-fiber fruits like apples, pears and cherries tend to have more fiber and lower glycemic indices. Other examples of "Life" carbs are whole grain breads, oatmeal and whole-grain cereals, whole-grain pastas, peanuts, wheat crackers, yogurt, milk, wild rice, vegetables and fresh or dried fruits, and beans (legumes).

Quick Energy Carbs: Some early research suggests that eating carbs during exercise gives athletes more energy.[21] **"Quick Energy" carbs are healthy, easily digestable (low to moderate fiber), and usually natural carbs with moderate to high glycemic indices.** (See "When You Should Eat" on page 39.) If you need to get energy for physical activity right away, eat these healthy carbs that release energy a little quicker (high glycemic index). Eat single-ingredient carbs (tropical fruits, pasta and sports drinks) instead of high-fiber foods (like bran) or foods with several ingredients (like muffins) which would be released even more slowly. In other words, healthy high-glycemic index carbs may be useful during and after workouts or matches. Tropical fruits like pineapples and mangoes have somewhat higher glycemic indices and lower fiber, and make decent Quick Energy carb sources. Other examples include sports drinks, watermelon, bananas, baked potatoes, graham crackers, waffles, "energy" bars, and honey.

Garbage Carbs: **"Garbage" carbs are usually low in fiber, have high glycemic indices, and often contain processed ingredients like the refined sugar in junk food.** Processing removes fiber and contributes to making a food into a "garbage" carb. ("Garbage" carbs are also called "simple" or "bad" carbs.) These are low in fiber and you can eat large amounts with a lot of calories and not feel full ("empty calories"). Garbage carbs get absorbed quickly causing a large, rapid insulin release, which may lead to increased conversion of calories into body fat and increased hunger later ("crashing and binging"). Avoid garbage carbs. If you are stuck eating these on occasion, be sure to eat small portions. Examples of "garbage" carbs include soda, white sugar, white bread, molasses, corn syrup, candy bars, ice cream, and alcohol (which your body converts to sugar right away).

> **Bottom line:** Life and quick energy carbs = energy! Avoid "garbage" carbs.

You should try to choose healthy carbs, and then ones with glycemic indices appropriate for what you need at the time. Remember: if you are going to experiment with high and low-glycemic index carbs, do it in the off-season or at practices, and not on competition days. See Appendix E: Carb Reference Chart on page 72 to compare different types of foods and the carbs they contain.

Normal adults require 130 grams of carbs a day, and athletes need much more depending on the intensity of their workouts. To calculate your carb requirements, multiply your weight (in pounds) x 3 or 4. That will be the number of grams of carbohydrate you should have per day. But depending on your workout levels you may need more. According to general population guidelines, carbohydrates should make up 45 to 65% of the total calories you consume. Some sports nutrition experts feel that they should make up 65% of your daily calories. One general guideline is: **carbs should take up about 2/3 of the plate at meals.**

Fiber

There are two types of fiber: Dietary and Functional. Dietary Fiber is the edible, nondigestible part of carbohydrates and lignin (another type of fiber) naturally found in plants. Good sources of dietary fiber are cereal bran, flaked corn cereal, sweet potatoes, fruit, vegetables, dried beans and peas, and oats. Functional fiber, which is gritty in texture, accounts for 70% of the fiber in our diets, mostly from wheat bran. Functional fiber has similiar health benefits as dietary fiber, but is extracted from natural souces or is synthetic. An example is pectin extracted from citrus peel and used as a food ingredient. The "Life" carb foods described above are usually high in fiber.

Fiber has many benefits for both wrestlers and the general population alike. Benefits of fiber include:

- ♦ It helps keep the digestive system regulated.
- ♦ It is filling without adding many calories. It can expand up to ten times it's size in the gut, providing a sense of fullness and satisfaction for a longer time.

- Fiber can give you an edge on weight management not only by helping satisfy your appetite but also by slowing the absorption of food. By providing slower calorie absorption, it prevents blood sugar from rising too rapidly and causing insulin surges which can lead to hunger in a little while. This way it helps sustain your energy levels throughout the day.

- It helps fat loss when it replaces fats and sweets. Fiber has fewer calories per gram (4 calories/gram) than fat (9 calories/gram) and is not easily converted to fat.

- Fiber may also help fight off some cancers, reduce risks of heart disease, lower cholesterol and helps prevent colon problems.

Try to have at least three grams of fiber per serving. Total daily recommendations for people under age 50 are 38 grams a day for males and 30 grams a day for females. Cereals, whole breads, brown rice, skins and peels of vegetables, and wheat bran are great sources of fiber. Whole foods are always better. For example, in some fruits and vegetables, most of their fiber is found in the skin. So there is more fiber in a whole apple than apple sauce, and there is none in apple juice. Be sure to check food product labels as some "high fiber" product labels can be misleading.

Fats

Fats have gotten a bad reputation because of their association with obesity and diseases. Everyone needs a little fat in their diets, and athletes are no exception. Fat is a good energy source for low intensity to moderate exercise, longer duration exercise, and may help prevent injury. (While athletes need some fat in their diets, it is not a great energy source immediately before a high-intensity exercise like a wrestling match.) Too little dietary fat may limit the duration of exercise and performance, and may affect muscles in certain ways. If your body is a car, think of carbs as the gas, but fat as the oil – a car needs some oil to run.

Most of the fat we consume is naturally found in foods (meats, nuts and dairy products) or added during the preparation of food (like fried foods). Sources of extra fat include margarine, peanut butter, salad dressings, oils, nuts or nut butters, mayonnaise, cream, chips, fried foods, fatty meats (bacon, sausage, pepperoni, bologna, etc.) Fat has nine calories per gram, where protein and carbs have only four calories per gram. So, eating less fat allows you to take in fewer calories without eating less food. According to general population guidelines, because fat has twice the calories of protein or carbohydrates, it should make up about 20 to 35% of the calories you consume. Some sports nutrition experts say fats should provide 20% of your daily calories, but others recommend the general guideline of the 35 to 40% range.

Eating too much bad fat is the easiest way to increase one's percent body fat, and excess body fat can interfere with performance in many sports. You may hear the term "fatty acid". This is just the basic unit of a fat molecule. The four main types of fat are made up of the different types of fatty acids.

The four main types of fat include:

Monounsaturated: These are liquid at room temperature and include canola, peanut oil, olive oils and most nuts. These are healthy fats that have a positive effect on cholesterol levels.

Polyunsaturated: These are soft or liquid at room temperature, and are found in corn, safflower, soybean and sunflower oils. They are also found in nuts and seeds. "Essential fatty acids" are polyunsaturated fats that our bodies need but cannot make on their own. These include Omega-3 fatty acids often found in seafood such as mackerel and salmon. These also have a lowering effect on cholesterol, but not as well as monounsaturated fats.

Saturated: These come mainly from animal sources like fatty meats (beef, lamb, veal, pork) and dairy products (butter, cheese, milk, cream), and anything containing hydrogenated oil. These bad fats are typically thick or solid. Avoid unhealthy saturated fats or "trans fats" like hydrogenated or partially hydrogenated fats. These include coconut oil (often used on popcorn at movie theaters because it smells so good), and vegetable shortening.

Trans Fats: These start out as unsaturated fats that undergo a process of hydrogenation to make them more solid like saturated fats. (Hydrogen is added to the fat molecule to make it more "saturated" with hydrogen.) This makes the fat more solid and extends its shelf life. This is the worst kind of fat, associated the most with diseases like heart disease.

The goal is to take in the right amount of fat, and try to take in healthy fats like those described here and in "How to Read Food Labels" on page 29. Good fats are the monounsaturated and polyunsaturated fats, and should be included to some degree in every athlete's diet. While you should watch how much fat you consume, you should not over concern yourself about fat intake! Fats are important for many body functions and add flavor and enjoyment to eating. Too much concern about fat intake may lead to too much weight loss and eating disorders, especially among teenagers. Such an "avoidance" of fat may cause teenagers to avoid foods such as red meat and dairy foods, which are important sources of many nutrients. Fat requirements: Desirable weight (in pounds) x 0.45 = number of grams of fat per day.

Protein

Athletes often think of protein in association with increasing muscle size and strength. In reality, protein is used for growth and repair of all the cells in your body and is very important for athletes, but it does not make you stronger. The average American eats twice the amount of needed protein each day, so you shouldn't need to worry too much about your protein intake. And most athletes eat more protein than they need. Protein shakes and supplements are unnecessary if energy needs are met by eating enough carbs and fats. In addition, they are usually expensive. (See "Protein and Amino Acid Supplements" on page 59.) Food is the easiest, cheapest, and best way to meet your daily protein needs.

Good sources of protein are meat, fish and shellfish, poultry, vegetables, eggs, grains, cheese, dry beans, soy products, milk or yogurt. *You do not have to rely on meat alone for good sources of protein.* There are many soy-based products and dairy products that are good sources of protein. Many plant foods like beans and nuts are good protein sources also. However, nuts are also high in fat and so should be eaten only in small amounts. According to general population guidelines, protein should provide 10% to 35% of your diet's calories. According to some sports nutrition experts protein should provide 15% of your daily calories.

One word of caution here: a recent study of wrestlers (*who were not practicing proper nutrition*) showed that they consumed a high-carbohydrate, low-fat diet but did not get enough protein. This deficient diet resulted in weight loss but also slowed the growth of their muscles. The result was decreased muscle strength during the season. Be sure you're getting enough protein in your diet. The recommended amount for the non-athlete adult is 0.8g per kilogram of weight or about 0.4g per pound of weight (about 25g a day for a 150 pound person). Teen athletes should consume from 0.8 to 1.0 g/kg/day. For an intensely training adult athlete it is between 1.2 to 1.5g/kg/day (0.6 to 0.8 gram per pound). Some experts push that number up to 2.0g/kg/day for adult athletes.

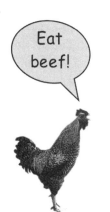
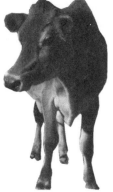

Vitamins and Minerals

Vitamins and minerals help your body "unlock" the energy in foods and help form building blocks for tissues in your body, but they do not provide energy themselves. Vitamins are complex substances found in foods that are vital to body functioning. There are a total of 14 vitamins, falling into two categories: water-soluble and fat-soluble. Water soluble vitamins include biotin, the seven B vitamins, vitamin C and choline. Fat-soluble ones include vitamins A, D, E and K. Minerals also fall into two categories: macrominerals and trace minerals. Macrominerals are ones that you need larger amounts of like calcium, phosphorus, magnesium, potassium, sodium and chloride. Trace minerals are neede in much smaller amounts. These include copper, iodine, iron, selenium, manganese, zinc and others. The term "electrolyte" refers to the minerals sodium, chloride and potassium when they are dissolved in your body, regulate chemical and water balances, and conduct electricity like that found in nerve signals.

If you eat a balanced diet from the basic food groups, you will consume all the vitamins and minerals your body needs. Eating enough fresh fruits and vegetables will help you get enough vitamins and minerals. (Remember, that's *fresh* fruits and vegetables — a number of vitamins are destroyed by air, heat, drying or aging.) Vitamin and mineral supplements are usually not needed, but if you really want to take a vitamin, choose a brand name multivitamin and mineral supplement that does not exceed 100% of the Recommended Daily Allowance (RDA) for each nutrient (like Centrum® or

One-A-Day®). [Note: Recently, the Food and Nutrition Board of the Institue of Medicine has released a new set of recommendations for the daily amounts of vitamin and minerals, called Dietary Reference Intakes (DRI's) and the Upper Levels (UL's) considered safe. These replace the previous RDA's.] Remember: don't get too much of a good thing. Some people mistakenly take too much of a certain vitamin and cause themselves additional problems. For example, too much vitamin A can cause osteoporosis in an older person, and too much magnesium can cause diarrhea.

Studies of active children and teenagers often identify a lack of two important minerals – iron and calcium. Calcium is necessary for development of bone mass and other body functions. Lack of iron causes anemia, impairs performance, interferes with muscle function and depresses brain function and motivation. Athletes need to be sure to get enough of these through proper diet. Female athletes who menstruate heavily should talk to their doctor to see if they need an iron supplement.

Sodium: an Important Mineral

For people with high blood pressure, heart disease or certain other medical problems extra salt (sodium chloride) can cause a lot of problems. So they need to carefully watch their salt intake. But because young, healthy, intensely training athletes lose much more sodium and chloride in sweat than any other electrolyte, they need to replace some of that salt. Sodium and chloride losses in sweat are usually less when an athlete is used to the heat and type/intensity of workouts. But some athletes may have more salt in their sweat than others, especially athletes beyond their teen years. As a lack of sodium can lead to incomplete re-hydration and muscle cramps, they may be more likely to get muscle cramps and may need a little extra salt in their diet. Salt and water tend to be absorbed together — to re-hydrate completely after exercise, you must replace the sodium and chloride lost in sweat. An extra shake of the salt shaker at lunch may help here — be careful as one simple shake of a salt shaker has a *lot* of salt in it!

> **Salt loss, muscle fatigue, conditioning and dehydration all play a role in muscle cramps. If you get muscle cramps often, a little extra salt in your diet may help.**[5] **(See WRESTLING HANDOUT #8: Muscle Cramps.)**

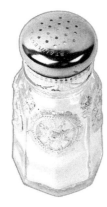

Be careful of some drinks with too much salt (like some vegetable drinks) as they may cause water retention prior to weigh-ins and competition. Salt tablets should only be used if you have repeated episodes of muscle cramps and *only if your doctor or trainer suggests them.* Also, drinking too much water too quickly when you are already low on sodium can cause dangerously low levels of sodium in the blood (called hyponatremia) which can be a very serious medical condition — this is more common in high-endurance sports like marathons or triathlons.

HOW TO READ FOOD LABELS*

"My doctor advised me to give up those intimate little dinners for four, unless there are three other people eating with me."
    – Orson Welles

Almost every boxed or packaged food now contains the Food and Drug Adminstration's Food Label (titled "Nutrition Facts") which lists its nutritional information. It tells you how many calories, how much fat, carbohydrate, sodium and other nutrients are in one serving of the food.

While the facts are shown on the label, you still have to read them and make your own decisions about how they fit into your nutritional goals. Learning to read labels will help you know the nutritional benefits or harms of a food. For example, some ingredients may not weigh a lot, but they can make a powerful difference, either good or bad, in your diet. The information on a food label is based on a 2,000 calorie diet. The following are key words for understanding food product labels.

- ◆ **Serving Size:** The serving size is how large your serving should be to get the amounts of nutrients and calories listed. If you double your serving size, then you will double the nutrients and calories. Be careful, as serving sizes can be smaller than you might expect. The serving size is based on the amount of food people say they usually eat in one sitting. This size is often different from the serving sizes in the Food Guide Pyramid.

  The portion size that you are used to eating may be equal to two or three standard servings. Look at this Nutrition Facts label for cookies. The serving size is two cookies, but if you eat four cookies, you are eating two servings – and double the calories, fat and other nutrients in a standard serving.

- ◆ **Servings Per Container:** The number of servings in the entire product or package. You may be surprised to find that small containers often have more than one serving inside. Learning to recognize standard serving sizes can help you judge how much you are eating. When cooking for yourself, use measuring cups and spoons to measure your usual food portions and compare them to standard serving

Nutrition Facts		
Serving Size 2 cookies (31g)		
Servings Per Container About 7		
Amount Per Serving		
Calories 110		Calories from Fat 20
		% Daily Value*
Total Fat 2.5g		**4%**
Saturated Fat 0g		**0%**
Polyunsaturated Fat 0g		
Monosaturated Fat 1g		
Cholesterol 0 mg		**0%**
Sodium 115 mg		**5%**
Total Carbohydrate 22g		**7%**
Dietary Fiber 1g		**6%**
Sugars 14g		
Protein 1g		
Vitamin A 0%	●	Vitamin C 0%
Calcium 2%	●	Iron 4%

*Percent Daily Values are based on a 2,000 calorie diet. Your Daily Values may be higher or lower depending on your calorie needs:

	Calories:	2,000	2,500
Total Fat	Less than	65g	80g
Sat Fat	Less than	20g	25g
Cholesterol	Less than	300mg	300mg
Sodium	Less than	2,400mg	2,400mg
Total Carbohydrate		300g	375g
Dietary Fiber		25g	30g

---

*The information in this section was adapted from information from the Food and Drug Administration, the National Institue of Diabetes and Digestive and Kidney Diseases [23], information distributed by the American Heart Association, from Mosby's-Year Book, Patient Teaching Guides [10] and from Global Health & Fitness.[11]

sizes from Nutrition Facts labels for a week or so. Put the measured food on a plate before you start eating. This will help you see what one standard serving of a food looks like compared to how much you normally eat. You do not need to measure and count everything you eat for the rest of your life – just long enough to recognize standard serving sizes. See the "Anywhere' Guide to Serving Sizes" on page 17.

♦ **Calories:** Knowing the number of calories in one serving will help you adjust your serving size. Watch this number carefully as even foods that are "nonfat" or "low fat" can be high in calories.

♦ **% Daily Value:** This is what fraction (or percent) of your total daily requirement is in a single serving. The recommended daily values (total recommended amount in a day) for vitamins are based on the U.S. Recommended Dietary Allowances (RDA's); meeting these values prevents vitamin deficiency diseases. (See the note on RDI's on page 28.)

♦ **Total Carbohydrates:** This is the weight of all types of carbohydrates (in grams) in one serving.

♦ **Fiber:** Fiber is divided into two categories: Dietary Fiber and Functional Fiber. Total Fiber = Dietary Fiber + Functional Fiber. (See "Fiber" on page 24.)

♦ **Sugars:** The weight of sugars (in grams) in one serving.

♦ **Protein:** Most products contain at least some protein. Be careful: while animal products contain protein, many also contain high amounts of fat.

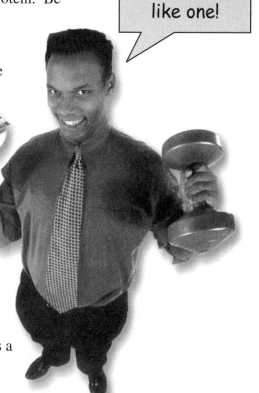

Eat a fish — don't wrestle like one!

♦ **Vitamins & Minerals:** Each product shows the percentage of your daily requirement of certain vitamins and minerals. Your diet should contain a variety of foods so that these add up to 100% every day.

♦ **Total Fat:** Your diet does not need much fat. Try to get your daily calories from products that contain little amounts of fat. Too many calories from fat may lead to heart disease and other health problems. The way to lower fat in your diet is to become a fat-conscious eater – and this requires that you know the amount of fat in each food. However, instead of counting fat grams and deciding if it is a "good food" or a "bad food," try to balance the foods you are eating so that you average 15 to 25% of your total calories from fat, depending on your body's requirements.

♦ **Saturated Fat:** Right below the "total fat" line is "saturated fat." Again, you want this number to be very low, since this type of fat is linked to higher cholesterol, obesity and heart disease. You should eat products that have little or no saturated fat. [Note: this part of the label will be changing in the near future. It will list the trans fatty acids which are fats that have no nutritional value and are even more closely linked to heart disease and obesity. They are also called hydrogenated or partially hydrogenated fats.]

♦ **Cholesterol:** Cholesterol is closely related to fat and may also lead to heart disease and other problems. Choose foods that have very low amounts of or no cholesterol. Your daily diet should contain no more than 300 mg of cholesterol.

♦ **Sodium:** Sodium is another name for "salt". For normal people the total daily intake of sodium should be no more than 2400 to 3000 mg a day. People with high blood pressure, kidney problems, water retention or heart problems need to watch their salt intake closely. But intensely training athletes may need extra sodium to replace that lost in sweat, and to help them re-hydrate well.

♦ **Daily Value:** This tells you the percentage of your daily allowance (RDA) that you are getting in one serving of this product. If you eat more, your personal daily value may be higher than what is listed on the label. If you eat less, your personal daily value may be lower. For fat, saturated fat, cholesterol, and sodium, choose foods with a low "% Daily Value". For dietary fiber, vitamins and minerals, your daily value goal is to reach 100% of each. For total carbohydrates, you may require more than the Daily Value depending on your training intensity level. If you have a 2,000 to 2,500 calorie diet, the Daily Values for total fat, saturated fat, cholesterol, sodium, carbohydrates, and dietary fiber are listed toward the bottom of the label. Eating amounts well above or well below these numbers on a regular basis can cause health problems.

♦ In addition to knowing how to read a product's nutrition label, you should know what the different terms on products mean. Below are terms that are often misinterpreted.[11]

♦ **Free:** As in "fat-free." The food has so little of the nutrient that it is not significant (usually less than 0.5 gram/serving).

♦ **Low:** As in "low-calorie" or "low-fat". The food has only a little of the nutrient, but enough to make a difference in your diet. More specifically, "low-fat" is three grams or less of total fat, "low-saturated fat" one gram or less, "low-cholesterol" is less than 20 milligrams, and "low-calorie" means 40 calories or less per serving.

♦ **Lean:** This means one serving of meat has less than 10 grams of total fat, four grams of saturated fat and 95 milligrams of cholesterol.

♦ **Extra lean:** One serving of meat has less than five grams of total fat and two grams of saturated fat.

♦ **Less:** There is 25% less of an ingredient or nutrient as compared to a similar product.

♦ **Reduced:** This means the product was nutritionally altered to meet a health claim.

- **Unrefined:** Always look for unrefined breads, pastas, cereals and flours. Refined grains have lost much of ther fiber, vitamins and minerals. The "enrichment" process only adds back a few nutrients. Look for the word "whole" as in "whole-wheat" or "whole-grain". Don't be fooled by the color of a food product. For example, some refined breads have molasses or brown sugar added to make them brown in color and appear whole. Oatmeal, brown or wild rice are always whole. White rice is refined.

- **USP:** This stands for U.S. Pharmacopeia. This has 18 standards for purity, quality and strength of vitamins and minerals. "USP" on a label means that the information on the label is accurate. Similar standards are presently being debated and developed for herbal products and supplements.

- **"Punch" or "drink":** For a drink to be labeled "juice," it must be 100% juice. If there is any added sugar it must be labeled "punch", "drink" or "cocktail". Do not buy drinks labeled with statements like "10% real juice" as they are 90% water and added sugar.

Check the List of Ingredients

Ingredients are listed in descending order according to their quantity. The first three or four ingredients listed usually make up most of the product. If an ingredient is listed fourth or fifth, it's amount is usually small. But be careful: an ingredient may be listed as one of the very last ingredients, but it is possible that the amount could be very high, even more than the total Daily Value.

Keep in mind that fat and sugar come in many different forms; even if they are not one of the first three ingredients, the food can still be very high in fat and sugar. Other names of fat include hydrogenated vegetable shortening, butter, margarine, oil (coconut, safflower, palm, etc.), lecithin, lard and cream solids. Other names of sugars include fructose, honey, corn sweeteners, molasses, maltose, corn syrup, fructose, galactose, glucose and dextrose. If only one of these names appears among the first few ingredients on the label, or if several of them are listed throughout the label, the food is likely to be high in fat or sugar.

Figure Out the Percentage of Calories from Fat

This is more important than simply knowing the number of grams of fat in the food. Just as you want 15 to 20% (and definitely less than 25%) of your total daily calories to be from fat, you also want to try to eat foods that get less than 15 to 25% of their total calories from fat. Because a food product has a low number of fat grams, it is not necessarily a low-fat food.

To calculate the percentage of calories from fat for a food do the following. Multiply the number of fat grams by 9 (there are 9 calories per gram of fat). Divide this number by the total calories per serving. Multiply this by 100 to get a percentage. This is the percentage of calories from fat (it should be less than 25%).

$$\% \text{ of calores from fat} = \frac{\text{fat grams per serving from fat}}{\text{total calories per serving}} \times 100$$

For example, in the macaroni and cheese Nutrition Facts label shown here there are 12 grams of fat per serving. So the amount of calories from fat in one serving is 12 x 9 which equals 108. There are 250 total calories in one serving.

The % of calores from fat = (108 ÷ 250) x 100 = 23.1%

Do not worry if you do not like math… estimating works. For example, if there are 100 calories and 25 are from fat, you could easily estimate the percentage of fat to be 25%. If the total calories are 120 (which is larger than 100), you can easily guess that it would be less than 25% fat.

Nutrition Facts

Serving Size 1 cup (228g)
Serving Per Container 2

Amount Per Serving

Calories 250	Calories from Fat 110

	% Daily Value*
Total Fat 12g	**18%**
Saturated Fat 3g	**15%**
Cholesterol 30mg	**10%**
Sodium 470mg	**20%**
Total Carbohydrate 31g	**10%**
Dietary Fiber 0g	**0%**
Sugars 5g	
Protein 5g	

Vitamin A	4%
Vitamin C	2%
Calcium	20%
Iron	4%

* Percent Daily Values are based on a 2,000 calorie diet. Your Daily Values may be higher or lower depending on your calorie needs:

	Calories:	2,000	2,500
Total Fat	Less than	65g	80g
Sat Fat	Less than	20g	25g
Cholesterol	Less than	300mg	300mg
Sodium	Less than	2,400mg	2,400mg
Total Carbohydrate		300g	375g
Dietary Fiber		25g	30g

Sample label for macaroni and cheese adapted from www.fda.gov

FOOD PREPARATION TIPS

Often, how foods are prepared can have a huge effect on both it's caloric value and appeal. Maintaining a variety of foods will help keep a healthy diet appealing and make it easier to maintain a positive outlook. Don't rely on a single food or food group to supply all of your needed vitamins and nutrients. Be creative. Don't be afraid to try new foods or experiment.

Make your kitchen and diet user friendly:

- ◆ Get good cutting boards, knives, measuring cups and spoons, salad plates, travel containers and nonstick cookware. Have them easy to get at.

- ◆ Make your refrigerator user friendly. Store precut carrots and celery sticks in clear containers on the top shelf. Keep low-fat condiments (like mustards, balsamic vinegar, salsa and soy sauce) near the front. Place water bottles in front of soda cans. Move tempting desserts or high-calorie foods to the back.

- ◆ Have healthy snacks handy in the kitchen like nonfat yogurt, frozen juice bars or "light" popcorn. Elsewhere, keep "travel foods" like sealed water bottles, nuts and fruit in your locker or bookbag.

- ◆ Make room on the counter for fresh fruits and vegetables. Get rid of the cookie jar, candy dishes, etc.

- ◆ Make dinners large enough for you to have leftovers the next day. Freeze restaurant leftovers so you are more likely to have them as a meal instead of a snack.

- ◆ Buy purified or spring water in plastic bottles. After you drink them, wash the bottles in hot, soapy water, refill them with filtered or purified tap water and keep them in the refrigerator for easy access. (Do not put them in the dishwasher.) Filtering or purifying tap water will improve it's taste and remove unwanted minerals and additives. Recycle or dispose of bottles when they get too old or worn.

- ◆ Buy some new healthy-eating cookbooks or get healthy recipes from the Internet. There are many websites offering countless free recipes.

- ◆ Encourage your family to be considerate – ask them to eat healthily when around you.

When preparing foods, try the following:

- ◆ Avoid fried foods and thick gravies. If you like the crispiness of fried foods, bake or broil non-fried foods a little longer (without burning it).

- ◆ Make favorite recipes with healthier ingredients. When baking, substitute half the fat with applesauce or trade some or all of the sugar with fruit puree or juice concentrate.

- Flavor with fat only in small amounts. Extra virgin olive oil packs a punch. Use a low fat oil spray instead of oil or butter when cooking.

- Use egg whites instead of whole eggs (the yolk of an egg contains most of the fat).

- Avoid high fat condiments like mayonnaise. Use nonfat yogurt in place of sour cream. Use pineapple, apple and orange juices instead of oil in salad dressings. Use lower fat condiments like ketchup, mustard, low-fat honey mustard, soy sauce, hot sauces or salsas.

- Use spices instead of fats to add flavor. Try fresh herbs instead of butter.

- Use low fat chicken broth, salsa, plain low-fat yogurt or fat-free cottage cheese to flavor a baked potato instead of using butter and sour cream.

- Try different greens in salads, like kale, romaine lettuce, field greens or baby spinach. These are often available packaged fresh in grocery stores. They are tastier and loaded with more nutrients. Try different things in salads for color and variety like garbanzo beans and cherry tomatoes.

- With pasta, use marinara sauce instead of meat sauce.

- Use good quality cheeses — they have more flavor, so you can use less of them.

- Remove the skin from chicken (this removes 2/3 of the calories) and all visible fat from meat. Choose white meat over dark meat (which has more fat). Choose lean cuts of meat and avoid fatty meats like hamburger and sausages.

Below are some ideas on how to make food healthier while keeping it appealing.

- Cook less often and eat more raw fruits and vegetables. For a snack during the day, take along cut veggies with low-fat dip. Eat a variety of fruits and vegetables — an apple every day will quickly get boring. Try mangos, sliced bell peppers, sugar snap peas, tangerines, grape or cherry tomatoes.

- Boil a dozen eggs and store them in the refrigerator for a quick and already prepared snack. Don't eat the yolks, as they contain most of the egg's fat and cholesterol.

- Make smart substitutions like unbuttered popcorn or baked potato chips for regular chips, canadian bacon for regular bacon, or an orange for orange juice.

- When craving a specific food, look for a low-fat alternative. Try to identify what it is about the food that you are craving. If craving something crunchy with a high salt content, try dill pickles instead of chips. Choose fruit when a sweet tooth acts up.

- Mix things up. Try adding fresh fruit to low-fat granola cereal. Try frozen fruit mixed with yogurt. Berry purées make great dessert toppings over sherbet or frozen yogurt.

- Try different types or flavors of juices and sports drinks instead of drinking only water.

- Be sure that foods taken to competitions are kept in coolers or refrigerated, or are foods or snacks that can be safely kept at room temperature like unpeeled fruit or pretzels. Don't eat leftovers that have not been properly refrigerated or are more than two days old – "when in doubt, throw it out".

DIET FOODS

Packaged diet foods like those sold by Weight Watchers®, Lean Cuisine® and Healthy Choice® are, in general, good alternatives. But be sure to read the labels carefully. Packaged foods are often too processed or refined to be as healthy as they claim to be. They may not be the ideal meal for a high-intensity athlete or growing adolescent. For example, some may be low in salt – inadequate salt intake for an athlete may lead to muscle cramps or other problems. Other products like some diet or sugar free candies may be high in sorbitol, which may cause problems like diarrhea when taken in large amounts.

Diet programs like Seattle Sutton's Healthy Eating™ can be very good because they follow nutritional guidelines very closely. *But they may not provide enough calories for the intensely training athlete.* Be sure to get enough calories along with the proper nutrients.

Beware of "diet" claims on packages. Read labels and pay attention to serving sizes. For example, don't pig out on "low-fat" cookies that can quickly pack on the calories. Also, reduced-fat or "lite" foods often have serving sizes smaller than their "normal" versions. (See "How to Read Food Labels" on page 29.) Also, food at fast food restaurants marketed as "lite" or "healthy" may not always be "lite" or "healthy".

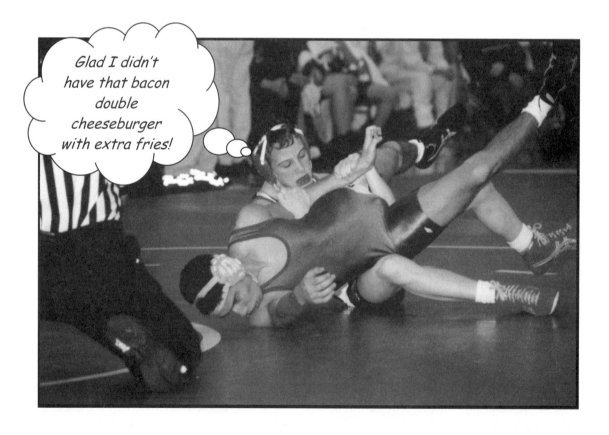

UNDERSTANDING HUNGER

"Thou should eat to live; not live to eat."
— Socrates

The most important thing about hunger and wrestling is: if you are managing your diet and nutrition properly, you should not be very hungry. But hunger may play a role if you have a lot of body fat to get rid of, especially while getting in shape during the off-season. If you understand where hunger comes from, it can be easier to manage.

Hunger and satiety (the satisfaction after eating) have several causes. Hunger is generally stimulated by low blood sugar. Satiety is mainly based on fat intake, and to some degree protein intake. Fat in the bloodstream is sensed by the body and creates the sense of "being satisfied" after a large meal. This is usually fully sensed about 20 minutes after eating. Ever wonder why they serve a high fat, high protein food like peanuts when you are on an airplane?

A sense of "fullness" in the stomach is created by the volume of food, and will last only as long as it takes the digestive system to move the food along the rest of the digestive tract. Some foods high in fiber expand their volume after being eaten and will help create a sense of fullness.

Cravings are triggered in relation to hunger itself, by psychological causes like emotional eating, by a deficiency of certain nutrients like iron, or by pregnancy. Aside from a normal liking of your favorite foods, healthy wrestlers shouldn't have many, if any, cravings.

Keep in mind that food choices can affect your performance, satiety, and ability to manage weight. Several factors affect your eating satisfaction and they are different from person to person. Some people find that eating an apple as a snack fills them up, whereas others do not. What's important here is to find a healthy eating style that is healthy and works for you. The more satisfied you are, the easier it is for you to stick to a healthy training and nutrition program.[27]

Tips to help manage hunger include:

- ◆ Foods with a lots of processed sugars are not as good for fending off hunger as those with natural sugars, like fruit and dairy products.

- ◆ To maintain a fuller feeling for a longer time, have a diet with good protein and lots of fiber. Protein-rich foods like meat, fish, and eggs provide a good level of satiety. Protein-rich foods that are low in fat provide the same satiety as high-fat, protein-rich foods. So choose the low-fat ones. Foods made with whole grains (high fiber) are better than those with refined grains. Whole fruits and whole breads will fill you up better than sodas or processed foods.

♦ Eat early and often – don't skip meals, especially breakfast! Frequent smaller meals and snacks (about every two or three hours) keep your metabolism burning throughout the day.

♦ Eat the most during breakfast, moderately at lunch, and lighter at dinner. If you are someone who doesn't like breakfast, bring a snack like a piece of fruit to eat later in the morning to get your body started. Eating lighter at dinner will make your weight loss easier and will help you sleep better. Depending on your schedule, avoid eating two hours before bedtime.

♦ Learn the difference between stomach hunger (when your stomach "growls") and mouth hunger (when you want something to chew or have a craving).

♦ Manage how your body handles calories. For example, eat snacks made up of different types of foods together like a combination of fruit, turkey, low-fat cheese and a piece of whole grain bread. Calories from different types of foods eaten together are absorbed and used at different rates and can help hold off hunger. Follow snacks with a glass of water.

♦ Feel how full you are. Try eating a small amount and then waiting 15 to 20 minutes to fully sense how full you are and how the food tastes before continuing to eat. Focus on enjoying the setting and your friends or family for the rest of the meal.

♦ If you eat and chew slowly you will taste the food more thoroughly. Pay attention to what you are eating and fully enjoy the smell and taste of your foods.

♦ Use your fork and knife as weight control tools. Cut your food as you eat it rather than cutting it all at once. Set your fork and knife down between bites.

♦ Use smaller bowls and plates – smaller portions will look larger.

♦ Take a standard serving out of the package and eat it off a plate instead of eating straight out of a large box or bag.

♦ Eat salads and vegetables first. Take seconds of vegetables or salads instead of high-fat, high-calorie parts of a meal such as meats or desserts.

♦ When cooking in large batches, freeze some food right away in single-meal-sized containers. This way, you will not be tempted to finish eating the whole batch before the food goes bad, and you will have ready-made food for another day.

♦ Eat at only one spot at home – no stand-up coutner eating, couch eating, etc. Avoid eating in front of the TV or while busy with other activities.

♦ Do not skip meals. It may lead you to eat larger portions of high-calorie, high-fat foods at your next meal or snack.

♦ Don't beat yourself up if you fail once in a while. Stay disciplined all week and allow yourself your favorite food at least once a week.

WHEN YOU SHOULD EAT

"Eat breakfast like a king, lunch like a prince, and dinner like a pauper."
    – Adelle Davis

First, there is no significant scientific data available regarding carb loading or "meal scheduling" in pre-teen athletes. Therefore, it may not be necessary or advisable for younger athletes to follow a strict diet/nutrition regimen, aside from favoring a healthy diet in general. One approach for parents would be slowly changing the pre-teen athlete's diet to a healthy one as outlined here, and being sure to meet caloric, hydration, protein and other needs for their age group. Additionally, they may try adding of a small amount of carbs to the young athlete's regular diet during the pre-season and watching carefully how well they do. If no problems arise, and other nutritional needs have been met by their regular diet, try slowly increasing carbs to meet their training requirements.

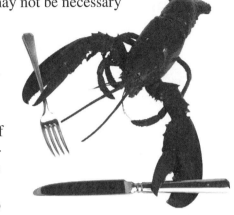

Teenage wrestlers may benefit from the nutritional information in this book because of being more physically similar to adult athletes. *The composition, amounts and timing of meals for teenage athletes should be carefully supervised.*

There are two main reasons why you should pay attention to when you eat. The first is to help maintain a healthy weight through proper eating habits, and the second is to maintain the right amount of energy supply for a high-performance athlete. For example, the above quote by Adelle Davis is true… for the most part. Eating a large breakfast does not necessarily help you eat less during the day but it does tend to make you more active and expend more energy throughout the day. It also helps ease hunger later in the day. Evening hours have a way of tempting people to overeat, so be sure not to snack for at least two hours before bedtime. But high-intensity athletes like wrestlers should focus on snacks and fluids at other times throughout the day to maintain a more even energy supply and avoid blood sugar "crashing", or having your body go into a "fasting state". Skipping meals can have negative effects on your performance by causing your body to use energy for daily functioning that would otherwise go towards training or competition. So *when* and *how often* you eat can be as important as *what* you eat both during the week and before and during competition.

If you spend a large part of the day starving and then trying to make up for it with a large meal at the end of the day, several things will happen. You will feel sluggish and lack energy for daily activities and workouts, you'll break down muscle proteins for energy, your blood sugar drops and you'll "crash" (get really hungry and be tempted to binge eat), and your body's "fat thermostat" turns on (causing your body to hang on to calories from a large meal eaten later in the day). Eating the right amount of calories but at the wrong time (like at the end of the day) will bring you back into "energy balance", but many of those calories won't be available for you to burn during the day and will consequently be stored as fat.

One key way of achieving and maintaining a healthy weight and body composition is by avoiding these large shifts in blood sugar levels (or the amount and size of these "energy swings"). Eating the typical three large meals a day forces you to eat a large amount of energy at only three meals. Staying in "energy balance" is easier when you eat frequent, smaller meals or snacks every three to four hours, breaking the standard three meals into five or six meals or snacks. This maintains a steady energy supply for your body throughout the day, helps control appetite, reduces binge eating, and keeps your body from going into the "starvation or storage" mode described above. But eating six meals a day is difficult with today's hectic schedules. One thing to try is to eat the three meals a day as you would anyway, but make them slightly smaller and definitely healthier. Then add two to three healthy snacks in between them. Examples of how to do this are found in Appendix B: Sample Meal Plans.

> **Eat a good breakfast and spread out your eating over 5 or 6 meals and snacks throughout the day. Frequent snacks and smaller to moderate-sized meals every 3 to 4 hours are better than starving all day and then eating a large, single meal.**
>
> **Eat most of your carbs and fats in the morning and afternoon. Carbs eaten during the day will provide you with energy to function well throughout the day. When these are eaten just before bedtime, they are not used right away and are more likely to be stored as fat.**
>
> **Remember: eating properly on the day of competition will not make up for poor nutrition during the week.**

Eating During the Off-Season

If you decide to experiment with your diet, do it during the off-season. Do not try to devise a "muscle diet" where you eat a lot of protein to pack on muscle. These do not work. Your body will build more muscle if it decides it needs it. (See "Protein" on page 26 and "Protein and Amino Acid Supplements" on page 59.) Instead, choose a generally healthy diet and work on establishing healthy eating habits and patterns so that when the season comes around, you can more easily focus on your "competition diet" as outlined below. Recently, 4,000 people on the National Weight Control Registry who lost 30 pounds and kept it off for at least one year were found to have four things in common that they did to lose and keep weight off. The purpose of mentioning this study is not to make you think that you have to lose a lot of weight and keep it off. But rather, take note of those four common things and keep them in mind when developing a healthy off-season lifestyle. People who are obese and lose weight do the best when they develop *healthy lifestyles*. The four things that these 4,000 people had in common were: they ate breakfast, they ate a low-fat/high-carb diet, they self-monitored (weighed themselves on a regular basis and did things like keeping a food diary), and they exercised regularly. Sounds a lot like wrestling, doesn't it? Another thing some people have found helpful towards living a healthy lifestyle include addressing emotional eating by finding support in people around them instead of food, and by thinking "What would I be feeling if I weren't eating?" Also, they stayed hydrated and cut down on alcohol. Bottom Line: during the off-season, focus more on eating healthy than on "dieting". Establish healthy eating patterns and habits so they are already in place when the season starts.

Eating Before and After Workouts

When deciding whether to eat or how much to eat before exercise, make the decision based on your energy level during your workouts. If you find yourself sluggish or running out of steam during your workouts, then you may need to take in more carbs. If your last meal was three or four hours before your workout, then you should eat a snack high in "quick energy" carbs (like whole bagels, crackers, fig bars, juice, granola or carbohydrate drinks) or a small meal within the 30 to 90 minutes before your workout.

What's more important is what you eat after your workout. After a workout, you will be thirsty and hungry and will be tempted to eat whatever you find. So it is important to have good, healthy foods easily accessible after practice. It is important to eat foods high in carbs with moderate amounts of protein within 30 minutes after a workout and eat a main meal about two hours after workouts. Doing this will help your body recover after workouts by replenishing energy stores (glycogen), and possibly improving muscle building/repair with protein if the food is eaten within 30 minutes of your workout's end. Not eating after your workouts makes the next day's performance harder because the muscles have not had a chance to reload with energy. Good foods for after workouts include: fresh fruit, bagels, raisins, sunflower seeds, yogurt, tuna, pretzels, low-fat granola bars, fruit juices, sports drinks and low-fat milk. Recommended guidelines are 0.3 to 0.6 grams of carbohydrate per pound of body weight (0.7 to 1.2 grams per kilogram), and one gram of protein for every three to four grams of carbs.

Think of eating for workouts in three parts: before, during and after workouts. Include "Life" carbs at each meal and "Quick Energy" carbs around workouts as follows:

♦ Before exercise, eat 50 to 100 grams of carbs 30 to 90 minutes before exercise. This will stimulate muscle glycogen storage and may help delay fatigue.

♦ During exercise, eat 30 to 75 grams per hour to help maintain training intensity. (As eating may not be convenient during a structured, two-hour wrestling practice, sports drinks may have a good role here.)

♦ After exercise – 75 grams of carbs within 30 minutes. This helps replenish muscle glycogen storage, especially within 30 minutes after the activity.

During the week do the following:

♦ **Eat or drink carbs before and after practices and matches. Eat a snack within 30 minutes after workouts and a full meal 1 to 2 hours after your day's main workout.**

♦ **Be sure to drink enough fluids throughout the day, and before and after practice (see "Hydration Guidelines" on page 45).**

♦ <u>**The bottom line**</u>**: Include carbs, protein (and some fat) at every meal. Have high-carb snacks at the proper times according to your workout schedule. Listen to your body, and notice how you feel and perform with eating changes.**

Eating Before Competition

Following proper nutrition and hydration practices will help you avoid any problems before training or competition. But you also need to individualize your "competition diet" according to your needs and your own digestion times and tolerances. Specifically, this means knowing how to supply the right amounts of energy from the sources you do well with, timing these properly relative to your matches, and avoiding foods that can cause problems. When developing your competition diet, consider making a food diary and noting how you do with different foods. Note how you felt prior, during, and after matches. Do not consider

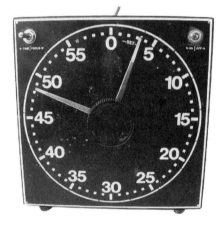

only whether you won or lost, but rather how well you wrestled and how you felt – and note that in the diary. In other words, keep perspective – do not discount the healthy foods you ate before you lost your match in the Olympic finals to Dan Gable. The "pre-competition time" should be considered the 24 to 48 hours before the meet, and your diet should be changed accordingly during this time. Do not experiment with new or different foods or supplements like sports shakes during this time – save that for the off-season.

♦ When you eat a regular meal, it takes about three hours for the food to be completely digested. You should eat a meal of easily digested foods at least three hours before competition. Avoid a meal that's too heavy or too light. If you do end up eating a heavy meal before competition, try to make it four hours before competition. If you eat a lighter meal, eat it two hours prior to competing. Eat a light snack 30 minutes one hour before competing.

♦ The more intense the competition, and the higher your anxiety level, the earlier the meal should be eaten. If you are too nervous to consume a lot of solid food before competition, you should eat frequent, smaller meals and eat softer, more easily digested foods like bananas, pastas and sports nutrition shakes. Some experts recommend meal-replacement drinks (like sports shakes) to minimize bulk in your stomach if your appetite is decreased in the hours before or after competition.[8]

♦   In general, it is best to start building your carb stores for competition by eating high-fiber, low-glycemic index foods (like apples) three to four hours before competition. Build into the "quick-release" good carbs (single-ingredient whole foods like baked potatoes and raisins) depending on how much time you have before competition.

♦   Make your pre-competition meals 2/3 (65 to 70%) easily digested carbs (low-fiber), and only about 1/6 of each of protein (10 to 15%) and fat (15 to 20%). Fats and proteins take longer to digest and can make you feel bloated prior to competition. Do not avoid protein and fats altogether, as you need some for proper body function, to decrease hunger, and provide a more long-term source of energy.

♦   Carbohydrate supplements ("energy bars") and liquid nutrition supplements can be taken up to one hour before training or competition, but you should experiment with such products to be sure that you do not have any problems. (See "Carbohydrate Supplements and 'Energy' Bars" on page 60.) Be sure that any nutritional supplements or shakes are cleared by your trainer, coach or family or team physician.

♦   Your weight should be under good enough control so that you can eat a good meal high in carbohydrates the night before competition. Some good ideas for "night before competition" meals include: pasta, pancakes, baked potatoes, breads and cereals.

Eating After Weigh-Ins

Things that may effect how well and how fast your body can recover after a weigh-in include the amount of weight lost, time allowed for recovery, methods of weight loss used, diet consumed during and prior to weight loss, and hydration and eating habits. This is why it is so important to practice proper nutrition and hydration in order to maintain a healthy weight near to or at your proper weight class. Then you don't have to "cut" weight before weigh-ins and cost yourself performance or strength.

After making weight, focus on foods and fluids that will help you recover and won't negatively effect your performance. Avoid bulky, fatty or seedy foods. Again, choose meals high in carbs with a moderate amount of protein and a little fat. Especially on competition days, carbs are easier on your stomach than a lot of protein or fat. High-fat foods are definitely slower digesting and may contribute to nausea during competition. Good competition day snacks are foods like pretzels, bagels, crackers, high-carb energy bars, fig bars, fruit, crackers, low-fat granola bars, applesauce, cereals and sports drinks.

During tournament days:

♦ **Eat a small snack and hydrate after weigh-in.**

♦ **Focus on hydration. Drink at least 2 cups of fluid within the hour before a match. Be sure to drink your needed amount of fluid throughout the tournament day.**

♦ **Do not skip meals. Eat frequent, smaller portions of high-carb snacks throughout the day.**

♦ **If eating a large meal, be sure it's at least 3 hours before competition.**

♦ **During a tournament do not wait for the entire round to finish and wait to eat as a team. Instead, follow the above guidelines acording to what *you* need and *when* you need it.**

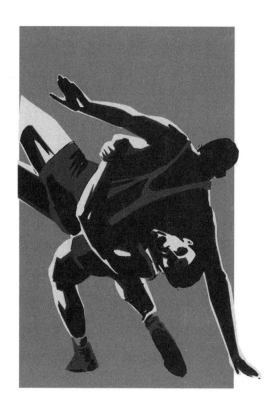

HYDRATION GUIDELINES

"Human beings are 70% water, and with some the rest is collagen."
        – Martin Mull

Maintaining proper hydration is difficult for people in general. An active athlete, whose requirements are greater, requires a conscious effort towards hydration. Traditionally, health experts have taught that eight 8-ounce glasses of water (64 ounces total) per day were needed to replace the daily fluid losses just from breathing, sweating and going to the bathroom. Although an old guideline, it is probably more than what most wrestlers are taking in daily. More recently, it's been recommended that an average, healthy, non-pregnant adult should consume one milliliter of water for every calorie burned throughout the day. For men that means about 12 cups, and for women nine cups. Those numbers increase drastically for the training athlete. (Follow the hydration guidelines on the next page and see "Dehydration" on page 51.)

The good news is that while drinking water is the best way to replace fluids, some of the fluids we need can be replaced by consuming certain solid foods and beverages. This includes milk, juices, sports drinks, and even fruits and vegetables. For example, cucumbers, lettuce and celery are 95% water.

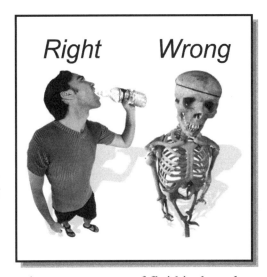

During physical activity, thirst is not a good signal of need for fluid. By the time you feel thirsty your body is already dehydrated. By the time you quench your thirst, you've replaced only about one-half to two-thirds of your body's fluid needs.

The best indicator of whether or not you are drinking adequate amounts of fluid is the color of your urine. Urine that is dark, concentrated or has a strong odor is a sign that you are dehydrated. Expect dark yellow urine after a practice or meet, but it should be clear before the next workout. Signs that your body is hydrated include moist mouth and lips, and moist eyes that easily tear. Also, you should be urinating every two to three hours.

Older guidelines stated that a wrestler can dehydrate up to 5% prior to competing; but it only takes a 2% loss of body weight due to fluid loss to result in reduced concentration and athletic performance. A 2% fluid loss is only three pounds for a 150-pound athlete!

Drinking plenty of fluids is the single most important thing you can do for good health and peak performance. Even a little dehydration can be a major cause of decreased performance, muscle cramps or heat illness.

Follow these important hydration guidelines:

- Weigh yourself before and after training to monitor fluid loss.
- Drink before, during and after practices and competition.

  ⇒ Drink 2 1/2 cups* of fluid 2 to 3 hours before training or competition and 1 to 2 cups of fluid 15 to 20 minutes before training or competition.

  ⇒ Drink every 15 to 20 minutes during workouts. You should have at least 1 cup of fluid every 30 minutes during workouts. If exercise lasts more than 45 minutes or is intense, consider a sports drink during the workout.

  ⇒ Drink 2 to 3 cups of fluid for every pound of body weight lost during exercise. This amounts to 150% of sweat loss (body weight loss) after exercise. Replace these fluids within 2 hours.

Also keep in mind:

- Drink early – remember to drink before you feel thirsty.
- Drink enough fluids during the day to have clear urine.
- One of the best ways to stay hydrated is to continuously drink smaller amounts of slightly cool water (between 50° and 60° F) throughout the day.
- Keep a log of fluid intake early in the season to be sure you are taking in enough fluids.
- If you are not used to drinking enough water before exercising, you will need to get used to it gradually. It may take a few weeks before you feel comfortable with this amount of fluid intake.

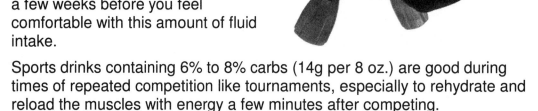

- Sports drinks containing 6% to 8% carbs (14g per 8 oz.) are good during times of repeated competition like tournaments, especially to rehydrate and reload the muscles with energy a few minutes after competing.
- To help speed rehydration consume foods and drinks that contain some salt (sodium) which helps the body keep more of the fluids.[8]
- Avoid drinks with alcohol and caffeine.

*one cup = 8 ounces

SAMPLE FLUID INTAKE LOG

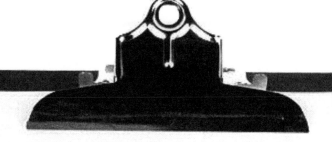

Wednesday, 12/10/03

7 a.m.	water 8 oz., sports drink 8 oz. morning run or weight lifting
8 a.m.	skim milk 8 oz., orange juice 12 oz.
10 a.m.	decaf cola 8 oz.
11 a.m.	skim milk 8 oz.
12 noon	bottle water, 16 oz.
2 p.m.	water 12 oz., sports drink 16 oz.
2:30 p.m.	wrestling practice -- weighed 150.4 #'s before & 149.0 #'s after practice -- lost 1.4#'s during

- drank water 20 oz., sports drink 16 oz. |
6 p.m.	skim milk 8 oz., water 16 oz.
9 p.m.	water 6 oz.
10 p.m.	lights out

EATING ON THE ROAD AND EATING OUT WISELY

"To me, an airplane is a great place to diet."
  – Wolfgang Puck

Today, Americans get about one-third of their calories from eating out, and they eat out twice as much as they did just a few decades ago. A typical fast food meal is high in fat and low in fiber and some vitamins. Be aware that you can eat half of your daily allowed calories in one meal if you are not careful. A large shake has over 1,000 calories, a blooming onion or an order of buffalo wings over 2,000, and cheese fries over 3,000! So the problem really is *fat food*, not fast food. Nothing is faster than grabbing a piece of fruit. It is difficult to choose a high-carbohydrate, low-fat meal at a fast food restaurant. But you can maintain your training diet when eating on the road or at a restaurant if you are careful about what you order. Examples of high-carb, low-fat meals at fast food restaurants are shown in Appendix C: Sample Restaurant Menus.

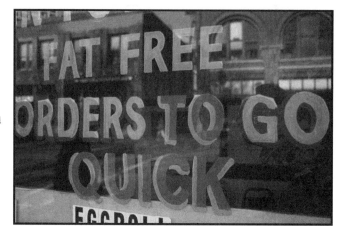

- Budget for more than just fast food. This will allow you healthier and tastier choices.

- Never go to a restaurant starving. Have a low-fat snack or glass of skim milk before you go.

- Pay attention to how foods are prepared. Choose food that is baked, broiled, boiled, roasted or poached. Choose foods served in a clear sauce (like *au jus*) instead of gravy. Avoid food that is breaded or fried.

- Do not be afraid to ask for food served "your way"; ask for extra vegetables on sandwiches, skip the extra cheese, request skim, low fat or 1% milk, and specify the topping you want.

- When ordering pizza, ask for vegetable toppings only and half the cheese.

- When you know you will be eating out, choose low-fat foods for your other meals that day.

- Fill up on low-fat items from the salad bar first. But avoid salad bar pitfalls like bacon bits, olives, cheeses and high-fat salad dressings. Also avoid mayonaisse-based salads like macaroni or bean salads.

- Choose fresh fruit or sorbets instead of unhealthy desserts. Bring fruit with you on the road.

- Eat your bread plain with a little olive oil or apple butter instead of regular butter or margarine.

- High fat foods in restaurants include ones with names like a la king, aioli, alfredo, batter-dipped, batter-fried, béarnaise, béchamel, breaded, carbonara, creamed, crispy, croquettes, fried, parmigiana and tempura.

- Order iced tea, sparkling water or low-fat milk instead of that milkshake. Ask for a slice of lemon in your water.

- Remove fat from foods like the skin on chicken, fat from meat and extra sauces.

- Request that a dish be made without a fattening ingredient or sauce, or have it served on the side.

- Getting a larger portion of food for just a little extra money may seem like a good value, but you end up with more food and calories than you need. Order regular-sized meals and drinks instead of "jumbo" or "super-sized". Keep in mind that "super-sized" soft drinks have a huge number of calories. Order the small size; choose a calorie-free beverage or low-fat milk. If you are with someone else, share the large-size meal. If you are eating alone, skip the special deal and just order what you need. (Remember: kid's meals usually come with a toy!)

- If you stop at a fast food restaurant, choose one that serves salads. Order single patty or smaller burgers. Eat the lettuce and tomato but scrape off extra mayo or sauce. Go without the cheese.

- Consider ordering the food you want "a la carte" or order two or three appetizers instead of a full entrée.

- Take half or more of your meal home. You can even ask for your half-meal to be boxed up before you begin eating so you will not be tempted to eat more than you need.

- Use the services of restaurants to your advantage. For example, if you see healthy foods on the menu prepared in unhealthy ways, ask them to prepare them in a different, healthier way.

- Be familiar with serving sizes of your favorite foods so you can estimate how much you are eating at an unfamiliar place.

- If faced with a vending machine, look for trail mixes, Rice Krispie Treats®, zoo crackers, pretzels, graham crackers or cheese crackers.

- If you go to the same place often and get to know the staff, your requests are more likely to be met. Tip well -- if you take care of the staff, they will take care of you!

- Make notes beforehand of restaurants or stores with healthy meals available in the cities where you are traveling.

- Pack wisely: be sure to bring a water bottle, cooler, ice packs, plastic silverware and trash bags.

- Remember… travelling may make you forget to stay hydrated. Keep focused on hydration especially when on the road!

When on the road, take along some healthy foods that won't spoil (nonperishable). A can of tuna or bag of pretzels packed with your gear as "back up" foods may give you added confidence that you have healthy alternatives if none are available. Bring foods like bagels or muffins, fresh or dried fruits, raw and cut vegegtables, unbuttered and air-popped popcorn, trail mixes, graham crackers, raisin bread, low-fat cheese sticks, fig bars, healthy cereals, low-fat granola bars, whole grain crackers, applesauce in sealed individual packages, and low-fat trail mixes. Zipper-type plastic bags make great travel containers. Bring along pastuerized/sealed packages of rice or soy milk, some cereal and raisins and you have an instant meal. Good ideas for travel drinks include juice boxes, sports drinks, decaffeinated iced teas and, of course, bottled water. Bring packets of powdered sports drinks for when you arrive at your destination. If your only option is soda, get one that is non-caffeinated.

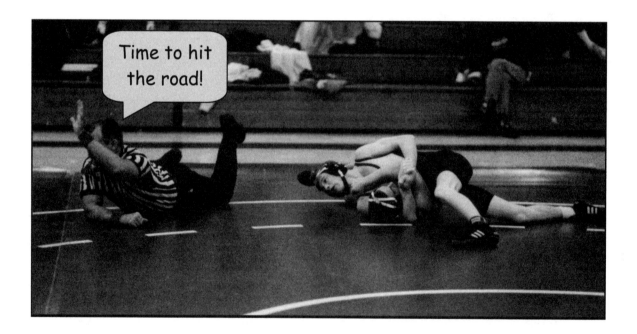

WAYS OF WEIGHT CONTROL TO AVOID

Wrestlers often use many ways to "cut" weight. Many of these have not always been the wisest things to do. Below are some of these and why they should be avoided.

Dehydration

Dehydration is loss of body water by not taking in enough fluids and/or too much fluid loss. Weight loss in wrestling that occurs in a short period of time consists primarily of water loss and should be avoided. A dehydrated body does not work as well. If you feel sluggish or fatigued, or if a practice or math "feels" difficult, you may not be hydrating enough or taking in enough calories. Athletes sometimes think feeling poorly like this means that they had a good workout when the opposite is true. A 1 to 2% loss of body fluids can result in a 15% to 20% decrease in performance![30]

Just like adults, children undergo progressive dehydration during exercise in a hot and/or humid climate. Kids' bodies do not regulate body temperature as efficiently as adults' bodies do. Dehydrating children would be more likely to suffer heat exhaustion and heat stroke earlier than adults would. Proper hydration is essential for the safety of active children. Consequently, younger wrestlers are more susceptible to heat illness. Heat injury, usually complicated by dehydration, is the second most common sports injury among kids, but is the most preventable.

> **When you rehydrate, your body absorbs water at a slow rate: only about two pints per hour, and it takes up to 48 hours for the water balance in your muscles to be restored.**

During exercise it is important to drink plenty of fluids, especially sports drinks or water. Dehydration can affect your performance in less than an hour of exercise -- sooner if you start the session dehydrated. A general guideline is to drink the equivalent of two to five 8-oz. glasses of fluids each hour of competition, depending on your size and training intensity level. A swallow of water is about 2 to 3 ounces. (See "Hydration Guidelines" on page 45.)

> **It is very important that you:**
> → **Limit weight loss by dehydration to a bare minimum, if at all.**
> → **Do not sit in a steam room or sauna to cut weight. (A sauna is a room with a temperature of 79º or above.) Do not exercise in vinyl, rubber or plastic suits. These practices are illegal as they can cause rapid dehydration leading to severe muscle breakdown and kidney failure (rhabdomyolysis), heart attack or heat stroke — all of which may be fatal.**

When dehydration results in fluid loss more than 2 to 5% of your body weight significant negative changes occur with exercise which may include the following:

→ **Decreased Muscle Strength and Endurance:** A decrease in blood flow to muscle tissues results in them working less well. Trying to use your muscles when you are dehydrated is like trying to drive a car without any oil.

→ **Decreased Heart Function:** With less blood and plasma volume, the heart works harder *and* less efficiently.

→ **Eye Trouble:** Dehydration can cause blurred vision and dry eyes.

→ **Reduced Nutrient Exchange and Acidosis:** With decreased blood flow to tissues, nutrients don't get delivered to the tissues, and the body's waste products do not get removed as quickly or as well. Also, acidosis occurs (a build up of acid which alters cellular function throughout the body).

→ **Heat Illness:** This takes on four forms: heat cramps, heat sycope (loss of conciousness), heat exhaustion and heat stroke – the last of which may be fatal. These result from an impaired ability to regulate your body temperature. Dehydration results in decreased blood flow to skin and muscles. The ability to sweat becomes compromised and core body temperature can and will rise. This increases the threat of heat exhaustion, heat stroke and severe dehydration to poorly hydrated athletes doing strenuous workouts. The danger is actually greater during a long practice workout in a warm wrestling room than in a match which lasts seven minutes or less.

→ **Decreased Kidney Function:** Low blood volume leads to decreased kidney blood flow and decreased kidney function. This contributes to the problems listed in the points here, in addition to decreased urine output, concentrated urine, and leakage of protein into the urine. It is not known if these changes can result in permanent kidney damage.

→ **Electrolyte Problems:** Decreased kidney function results in imbalances of electrolytes such as unhealthy increases in potassium and sodium.

→ **Mood Swings and Mental Changes:** All of the above contribute to increased mood swings, poor concentration and focus, disorientation and other mental changes.

Wrestlers "drift", or lose ½ to two pounds overnight, and wrestlers should know exactly how much they drift. They should take this into account when planning how much to drink the night before a weigh-in.[9] Older wrestling rules allowed up to five hours between weigh-in and competition – a wrestler could dehydrate up to 5% of his body weight and still have significant time to recover. Under the new rules, there is only one to two hours before competition and you should not dehydrate more than 1 to 2%, if at all, because there will not be enough time for your body to physically recover in time for competition. If you choose to not drink much the night before a competition, this should be a short-term and easy "drift" dehydration, that is, with little effort and *only* overnight before the weigh-in.

Some wrestlers can tolerate more dehydration better than others. So coaches and parents need to be wary of the wrestler who decides that he can dehydrate because he or she thinks they can "tolerate" it.

Factors negatively affecting an athlete's ability to tolerate dehydration include:

- ◆ Poor fitness levels

- ◆ High body fat percentage

- ◆ Less of a "natural ability" to tolerate dehydration

- ◆ Medications, illness or fevers

- ◆ Not hydrating properly (See "Hydration Guidelines" on page 45.)

- ◆ A workout environment that's too hot or humid (like some wrestling rooms)[12]

- ◆ Too much clothing (like extra sweats), or obstructive clothing (like rubberized suits)

If a wrestler is unwise enough to use saunas, plastic-type suits, laxatives or other unhealthy methods of dehydration or weight loss, it is also the parents' and coachs' responsibility to do their best to step in and stop it, even if it means removing that wrestler from the line-up.

Fasting

When you do not eat at all (fasting), your body uses its stored nutrients and weight loss will result. However, the body looks for sources of energy other than fat and finds it in muscle proteins and glycogen.

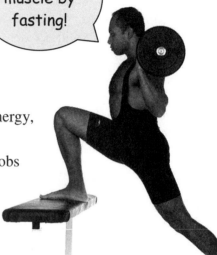

The bad effects of fasting include:

- It causes your body to use muscle proteins for energy, even if fat is available.

- It quickly lowers your blood sugar, which then robs your brain and muscles of their energy.

- It causes your body to lose large amounts of water, electrolytes and minerals.

The above effects undermine your strength and endurance in addition to robbing your body of needed energy stores you'll need later for competition. Eat at least *the minimum* calories your body requires each day so you can maintain your energy and strength while losing weight.

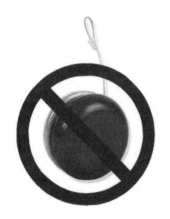

The greater the peaks and valleys in your weight, the more difficult it is for your body to function correctly. When your body goes from a starving state to suddenly eating a lot it hangs on tightly to each calorie to prepare for the next "starve" it may encounter. With each fast your body lowers it's metabolism and "gets better" at storing fat to prepare for the next fast. This places a big stress on your body and also makes losing weight more difficult. This is sometimes called "yo-yo" dieting. Don't be a yo-yo.

Avoid "semi-starvation" diets – those in which the number of calories you consume during a 24-hour period is more than 500 to 1,000 below the number of calories you burn. Losses greater than 500 to 1,000 calories a day usually result in very little additional fat loss and promote water and muscle loss.

> **Eating frequent small meals and snacks is much better than skipping meals or fasting.**

Fad Diets

Fad or extreme diets only result in short-term weight loss, usually do not consider the other aspects of nutrition needed by athletes, and are not as good as healthy diets. For example, low carbohydrate diets may result in weight loss in non-athletes by decreasing the amount of insulin the body produces in response to carbohydrates, and consequently less calorie "absorption". These diets promote protein and fats at the expense of carohydrates. *So they do not supply the amounts and types of energy needed for intense training. These diets have not been proven safe in the long term and are not recommended for athletes.*

The average American eats too many simple carbs like processed sugar, white flour, and alcohol. Because these are so low in fiber, people tend to eat large amounts of them without feeling full. Also, these high-glycemic index carbs are absorbed quickly, causing blood glucose spikes that lead to insulin surges. This can cause blood sugar levels to drop, causing even more hunger. When people go on a high-protein/low-carb diet, several things may happen. Any weight lost in the first few days or weeks of an extreme or fad diet is usually from dehydration and snaps right back. They may lose weight *in the short term* by restricting calories by cutting back on typically eaten *simple* carbohydrates. Also, they may take in fewer calories by cutting back on the insulin surge/hunger cycles associated with simple carbs.[26] Unfortunately, their intake of fat and fat calories may soar if they choose high-fat protein foods in place of low-fat protein or carbs. <u>The bottom line is that this type of weight loss is only a short-term phenomenon – real weight loss that stays off is due to lifestyle changes and healthy eating. The key to a proper diet is not to go from simple carbs to high-fat, high-protein foods such as fatty meats – but instead switching from "garbage" carbs to complex carbs (high-fiber or whole foods) such as fruits, vegetables, beans and whole grains, and switching from high-fat foods like salami to low-fat foods like fish or poultry.</u>

Diet Pills, Diuretics, Laxatives and Emetics

When used for weight loss in wrestling, diet pills, diuretics (water pills), laxatives and emetics (drugs that make you vomit) will dehydrate you and rob your body of important nutrients. Diet pills can have many bad physical and mental effects like causing mood swings, insomnia, or raising blood pressure. Laxatives and emetics can cause serious stomach and intestinal problems when used wrongly. Using these for the purposes of weight loss is just plain stupid.

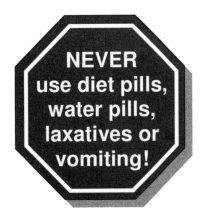

Nicholas Rizzo, M.D.

EATING DISORDERS AND WRESTLERS

Eating disorders are illnesses and are usually a type of coping stragegy that someone uses to deal with deeper problems too painful for them to handle directly. Eating disorders are often expressions of a need for control – a substitution for lack of control the person may feel in other areas of his or her life. Often, eating disorders are a cry for help. This is why trying to trick or force someone to eat can make things worse, as it is not the answer they are seeking.

Approximately 6% of wrestlers meet the criteria for binge eating, 10% meet criteria for eating disorders, and up to 45% of younger wrestlers may be at risk for eating disorders. *But this does not necessarily mean that they have eating disorders.* Rather, they may more likely have "disordered eating". After the wrestling season ends, most wrestlers resort back to "normal" eating habits. This suggests that this "disordered eating" is done with a conscious intent toward being fit for a sport, *and not as a result of the unhealthy causes associated with eating disorders.* This does not mean that eating disorders are not seen in wrestling – they are, just as in any other sport. *Be aware that eating disorders can be contagious and can spread through a team, and may include weight gain and weight loss. Nutrition, low body fat percentage and body image are issues of concern for male and female athletes in any age range.*

While eating disorders are more often seen in young women, all coaches, parents and teammates should keep an eye out for and bring attention to potential eating problems. Keep in mind that not every eating disorder is anorexia. Many student-athletes struggle with food, weight, and/or body image concerns. These may result in restrictive dieting, emotional overeating, compulsive exercise, use of weight loss products or harmful nutritional supplements, cigarette smoking, or excessive caffeine consumption. For example, male athletes are more and more exposed to "super male" images like professional athletes, magazine covers and television ads, and they may become increasingly unhappy with their appearance. This can be associated with a psychological problem called "body dysmorphic disorder", which is the preoccupation with an imagined or slight defect in one's appearance. Another example: in female athletes the combination of weakened bones (osteoporosis), absence of menses (amenorrhea), and eating disorders, along with delayed physical maturation, has been associated with excessive weight loss and sports participation at weights below minimum natural weight.[2]

A word of caution: Weight loss in young children (that is, before puberty) should be done very carefully. Unhealthy patterns of weight loss such as weight cycling, too rapid or excessive weight loss, eating disorders, excessive restriction of calories, or poor nutrition during these important growth years can have a negative effect on adult height and health. This can lead to impaired growth, strength and endurance. While hormone shifts have been described at low body fat percentages both in wrestling and other sports (such as lower testosterone levels in men and absence of menses in women), there is little evidence supporting long-term stunted growth or other problems *when healthy, responsible weight management is practiced.*

Below are some suggestions that coaches, parents and teammates should follow with regard to the athlete with an eating disorder. These should be a start only, and are not a complete answer – leave short and long-term treatment to professionals in this area.

♦ Be educated about eating disorders and know warning signs such as poor performance, mood swings, depression and social withdrawal, odd or avoidant behaviors, insomnia, eating in isolation, compulsive exercise, continual dieting (although thin), fear of weight gain, fatigue, significant weight loss, binge eating, vomiting or purging, abuse of laxatives and diuretics, brittle hair and nails, irregular or absent menses, heartburn or bloating, dental problems, reddened fingers from induced vomiting, etc.

♦ Recognize how powerful an eating disorder is – remember that it is an illness.

♦ Have a plan ready in case suspicious behaviors arise. *Know who to talk to right away.*

♦ Avoid commenting on appearance. Comments about weight, appearance or target weight classes (even if your intention is complimentary) will only reinforce their obsession with body-image. Avoid comments like "You look like you've lost weight", or "You need to lose five pounds this week."

♦ Realize that when approached about an eating disorder, a person may react with anger or denial. They may only discuss their eating disorder when they feel ready. They may feel more comfortable if they know that you are not going to force them into anything before they are ready (an exception may be if the condition is a medical emergency). *It may be necessary to pull an athlete from the lineup until medically cleared by a psychiatrist experienced with eating disorders.*

♦ Be prepared for the possibility that a discussion about their problem might not lead to a change in attitude or behavior on their part. This is because the person may have very good reasons for not giving up the eating disorder as a "coping strategy".

♦ Set a good example by your own behaviors involving food and exercise.

♦ Be compassionate *but do not take on the role of a therapist.* Leave that to a therapist.

♦ Admit your anger, frustration, and helplessness – but don't take it out on the person. It is often helpful for family or friends to get some support for themselves like seeing a licensed counselor or therapist.

♦ Support healthy nutrition through the consumption of a variety of foods rather than reliance on nutritional supplements.

If there is a question of an eating disorder, emotional or psychological problem, talk to a physician and mental health professional immediately.

For more information:

Anorexia Nervosa and Related Eating Disorders Inc., www.anred.com

The National Eating Disorder Information Centre, CW 1-211, 200 Elizabeth Street, M5G 2C4, Toronto, Canada, Toll-free 1-866-NEDIC-20 (1-866-63342-20), www.nedic.ca

The National Eating Disorders Association, 603 Stewart St., Suite 803, Seattle, WA 98101, Telephone (206) 382-3587, www.nationaleatingdisorders.org

NUTRITIONAL SUPPLEMENTS

Nutritional supplements (sometimes called "fat burners" or "muscle builders") include substances like creatine, androstenedione ("andro"), ephedra (ma huang), ginseng, yohimbine, smilax, tribulus, wild yams, gamma oryzanol and protein supplements. Despite what the labels or your friends may say, *many supplements come with risks and there is no scientific study that shows any benefit in competition. Large doses of supplements do not make up for a lack of training or ability, and some may be very dangerous.*

Serious mistakes people make about supplements include:

♦ Parents and coaches may advise wrestlers to take supplements to gain athletic ability by physically maturing faster, and thereby improve performance. However, physical maturity and athletic ability do not necessarily depend upon how early a young athlete reaches adolescence, and physical maturation will not be positively affected by any supplements. What's more concerning is that this may delay or stop the young athlete's normal growth.

♦ Some athletes may feel a false sense of security because they are taking supplements, and this may lead to poor eating habits. Athletes may think that their morning dose of supplements provides them with all of the nutrients and energy that they need, so that they end up eating whatever they want throughout the day. The result is poor nutrition and poor performance.

♦ The athlete may mistakenly associate perceived improvements in performance with whatever supplements they may be taking at the time (placebo effect). They may be less likely to attribute any progress to training, hard work and proper nutrition − the things that really do make the difference.

♦ Don't confuse an altered mental state or mood with performance. For example, ephedra may make you feel energized, but it does not provide additional energy. It is banned by several sports governing bodies and has been associated with the deaths of athletes.

Serious physical problems of some supplements include:

♦ Raised blood pressure	♦ Kidney problems
♦ Rapid heart rate	♦ Liver damage
♦ Nerve paralysis	♦ Seizures
♦ Dehydration	♦ Mood swings
♦ Diarrhea	♦ Loss of sleep (insomnia)
♦ Sweating	♦ Interactions with medications
♦ Coughing	♦ Stroke
♦ Stomach problems	♦ Death
♦ Increased bleeding time	

Nutritional supplements should not be taken. These are not regulated by the FDA like prescription medications or foods and may be harmful or dangerous. Supplements cannot take the place of healthy nutrition and proper training. (A brand name multivitamin like Centrum® taken once daily is okay.)

Beware:

- The ingredients listed on the label may not be the only ingredients. They may include anabolic steroids, caffeine, ephedrine and other substances.

- The ingredients may not be present in the amounts stated.

- Claims that herbal ingredients like yohimbine, gamma oryzanol or others can build muscle and improve performance have little or no scientific proof.

Note*: A few years ago an Olympic wrestler was barred from competition for two years after testing positive for the steroid nandrolone. He unknowingly took the anabolic steroid in a diet supplement that did not list the drug in its ingredients.*

Another Note: *Just because a supplement is available on the Internet does not mean it's safe. For example, ephedra (which has been associated with several deaths) has been banned by the FDA for sale in the U.S. Just because its possible to get it online from companies overseas does not mean it will not hurt you.*

Steroids

Steroids or anabolic steroids are *not* allowed in the sport and may do serious harm like weaken tendons or cause liver failure. <u>Warning</u>: these may be found in some nutritional supplements as described above.

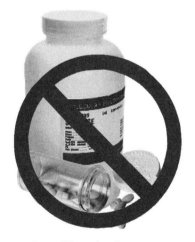

Protein and Amino Acid Supplements[19]

Proteins are simply chains of amino acids. Amino acids are simply the building blocks of a protein. So you can think of protein supplements and amino acid supplements as being essentially the same.

Many athletes think that extra protein helps them build bigger muscles. Your body gets more than enough protein for muscle growth and repair from a healthy diet – extra protein is either used as energy or stored as fat. In other words, extra protein just ends up as extra calories. It is easier, cheaper and safer to simply eat more carbs as your main energy source for strength training, and that will save the protein and amino acids in your regular diet for muscle building. Protein is protein – that is, protein from a supplement acts the same in the body as protein from food. Where do you think they get the protein in supplements from? Food! One 3-ounce serving of poultry or fish, two servings of low-fat yogurt, 4 eggs, or one serving of refried beans has as much or more protein than most expensive protein shakes and each of these is a lot cheaper! While a small amount of protein combined with good carbohydrates is recommended within 30 minutes of a workout, this does not mean you should eat the big protein loads in many protein supplements (See "Eating Before Competition" on page 42).

No benefit has been shown in athletic competition from using protein supplements, amino acid supplements (the building blocks of protein) or branched-chain amino acids (BCAA's). Taking in large amounts of certain amino acids can impair the absorption of other essential amino acids and have a negative effect on your health and performance. In addition to usually being expensive, they may possibly cause kidney problems, dehydration (by causing increased urine output), stomach upset and diarrhea.

Carbohydrate Supplements - "Energy" Bars and Sports Gels

These bars are often packed with lots of protein, vitamins, minerals and carbs. But there is no proof that there is anything special about these bars. Do not be misled into thinking that the word "energy" means that it will make you feel more energetic. The word "energy" is just another name for "calories". These bars do not improve athletic ability, and are much more expensive than other carb food sources. These bars are often marketed with different "goals" in mind, like "energy" or as "high-protein muscle-builders". Basically, these just have different amounts of carbs, protein and fat. High-carb bars (70% of the calories from carbs) are not bad. If you follow a proper diet, there should be no need for high-protein bars. Be careful, as some of these bars can have as much as fat and calories as a candy bar.

They do have some advantages though. They can provide extra carbs if you feel you need more energy/calories (despite a proper diet) after workouts or during competition. Another advantage is convenience. For example, some athletes use them as a convenient food source that is easy to carry, especially during long competition days or while on the road. If you feel nervous before competition and do not want to eat much, carbohydrate energy bars are a good alternative. If you are craving junk food like a candy bar, have an energy bar instead.

You can make an equally good "energy snack" for a lot less money, like combining granola or oatmeal, raisins, honey, a granola bar or a whole-grain bagel one hour before exercise. If you really want to use these, find one low in saturated fat and with an appropriate calorie amount. Read the labels, as you may be better off with the bagel or low-fat granola bar.

Sports gels (sometimes called "Carb Loaders") are quickly absorbed carbs in a gel form, kind of like an energy bar without the other nutrients. Gels are more commonly used in long endurance sports like marathons. Refer to the paragraph "Carb Loaders" on page 21.

Bottom Line: "Energy bars" are not magic. However, you can use them for convenience or as carb supplements on competition days, and only if you feel you need more carbs. Read their labels closely. You need to drink plenty of fluids if you eat energy bars or sports gels.

Creatine

Creatine has been shown to enhance short term high-intensity activity, but has not been shown to be of benefit in the more intense sports like wrestling. It does not make your muscles bigger, and it does not make you stronger. Creatine just "soaks up" water in your muscles and they feel bigger. In reality, this water just weighs you down and may cause problems when weighing in. Furthermore, because this water is "soaked up" with the creatine, it is not available for your body to use (called "intravascular dehydration"). This does not help you in any way and may contribute to dehydration.

Creatine may cause:

- abdominal pain
- intestinal problems
- kidney problems
- dehydration
- weight gain by retaining water

Creatine has not been shown to be of any significant benefit in the more intense sports and has no role in wrestling.

Over-the-counter Vitamins and Supplements

While certain vitamins are proven to help certain illnesses, most scientific evidence does not show that vitamins or supplements will improve performance for young athletes (for example, gingko biloba, garlic, fish oil, vitamin E, vitamin C, etc.) There are reports of glucosamine/chondroitin helping older people with joint pain, but results from large scientific studies are not yet complete, and this has not been evaluated in athletes. Some of these will interact with certain prescription drugs and over-the-counter medications. In addition, too much of a vitamin or mineral could be harmful. For example, too much vitamin B-6 can cause nerve problems. See "Vitamins and Minerals" on page 27. A once daily brand name multivitamin is acceptable.

CAFFEINE

"Resolve to free yourselves from the slavery of the tea and coffee and other slop-kettle."
– William Cobbett, <u>Advice to Young Men</u>, 1829

Caffeine has been shown to help athletic performance only:

- ♦ when taken in small amounts (one to two cups)
- ♦ in long endurance types of sports like marathons
- ♦ when the athlete does not drink a lot of it on a daily basis

<u>Note</u>: none of the above conditions apply to wrestling.

So, while it may *seem* to help athletic performance in the short term, other studies show no consistent benefit, no benefit in someone that already drinks three or more cups of coffee a day, and no benefit in shorter-duration and strength-oriented sports like wrestling.

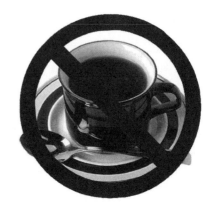

Effects of too much caffeine include:

- ♦ jitters and tremors
- ♦ irritabilty and anxiety
- ♦ rapid or irregular heart beats
- ♦ clammy hands
- ♦ upset stomach
- ♦ fatigue
- ♦ increased appetite
- ♦ diarrhea
- ♦ dehydration
- ♦ decreased sleep

If you drink a lot of caffeine and stop too quickly, you may experience caffeine withdrawal headaches. Switch to decaf gradually.

<u>**Bottom line**</u>**: As caffeine offers no real benefit to wrestling and it causes dehydration (even in small amounts), the serious wrestler should not drink caffeine often if at all – certainly no more than one cup of coffee in the morning, and that only if you absolutely need it.**

TOBACCO, ALCOHOL and ILLEGAL DRUGS

"If we burn ourselves out with drugs or alcohol, we won't have long to go in this business."
– John Belushi

Tobacco, alcohol, and illegal drugs have no role in wrestling. Alcohol, tobacco (chewed or smoked) and illegal drugs (marijuana, cocaine, ecstasy, etc.) are harmful in many ways. While some people may say that some of these may "calm them down", in reality they increase the stress on the mind and body by decreasing performance and concentration.

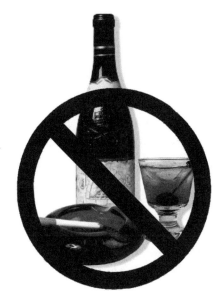

Tobacco, alcohol, and illegal drugs all do at least one or more of the following:

- ◆ Decrease conditioning, strength and reflexes
- ◆ Increase risk of injury and illness
- ◆ Cause dehydration
- ◆ Raise blood pressure
- ◆ Cause blood sugar to drop too low
- ◆ Deplete essential nutrients and energy
- ◆ Cause mood swings and loss of sleep
- ◆ Cause problems at school or work
- ◆ Interact with prescription and over-the-counter medications

In addition, these are either illegal or have minimum age requirements. Tobacco, alcohol, and drugs are against most school rules and may be grounds for expulsion or suspension from extracurricular activities and athletics.

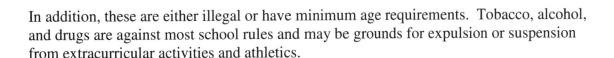

Care about yourself and your wrestling – do not put yourself at a disadvantage by taking the risks that come with using alcohol, tobacco or illegal drugs.

<u>BRINGING IT ALL TOGETHER</u>

"Respect all. Fear none."
   – Anonymous

Being a champion means doing your best in all aspects of the sport. In wrestling, that includes good technique, proper training and conditioning, the right methods of weight control, good nutrition, staying hydrated, staying healthy and showing good sportsmanship. In addition, taking care of yourself physically, mentally and academically will reduce stress and make you a better wrestler and student.

It also means doing the following:

- If you have any medical conditions (like asthma), discuss the proper treatment with your doctor, both in general and as it relates to the sport of wrestling. See your doctor if needed. Don't wait thinking that a problem "will just get better".

- Inform your coaches if you have any medical conditions or are taking *any* prescription drugs or over-the-counter medicines. Some over-the-counter medicines like pseudoephedrine are against the rules in some international competitions.

- Tell your parents and coaches when you have an illness, skin rash, injury or other problem. This includes trouble in school and problems with peers. These may affect you and your wrestling.

- Be sure to get eight hours of good rest each night. Your body uses that time to rebuild and refuel. Sleep has also been shown to have an effect on weight control, energy and ability to concentrate throughout the day. Getting enough solid rest is crucial to your success.

- Manage stress appropriately, especially if it is affecting your sleep.

- On and off the mats you represent your sport, school, coaches, teammates, parents and yourself. The best athletes do not have unsportsmanlike conduct or rude behavior — a victory is not a true victory unless it is received with honor. Good sportsmanship means no showing off – whether you win or lose come off the mat quietly with class. Even if you win a big match, you should act like you've "been to this barbeque before" and you were just doing what you were supposed to do.

- Most importantly, being a responsible wrestler means that you are a responsible student. If your grades are suffering then you are not achieving your goals as a student-athlete.

- Respect yourself by respecting others and by achieving your best. Use the tools of character, discipline, and self-knowledge that the sport of wrestling gives you to be a champion in all aspects of your life.

If you do all of the above, you'll wrestle better knowing that you have done *everything* possible to be at your best.

APPENDIX A: How to Estimate Your Minimum Wrestling Weight and Appropriate Weight Class

Today, the way to determine your appropriate wrestling weight that is most reliable and still convenient is to have skinfolds performed by qualified personnel, and then have those values entered into the NWCA Weight Certification Internet Calculator Program, as described in the section "Weight Class Certification" on page 6. If you do not have internet access, you can use the following calculations to estimate things for your own knowledge and at least be familiar with the math and concepts.

To Calculate Your Fat Weight:
  Have your percent body fat determined through skinfold measurements. Multiply your weight in pounds by your percent fat (as a decimal). For example, if you weigh 140 lbs. and are 12% fat:
    140 x 0.12 = 16.8 lbs of fat

To Calculate Your Lean Body Mass:
  Subtract your fat weight from your body weight:
    140 - 16.8 = 123.2 lbs. of lean body mass (LBM)

3. To Calculate Your Minimum Wrestling Weight:
  For males at 7% body fat: divide LBM by 1 minus that percent (1 - 0.07 = 0.93):
    123.2 ÷ 0.93 = 132.5 lbs.

  For females at 12% body fat: divide LBM by 1 minus that percent (1 - 0.12 = 0.88):
    123.2 ÷ 0.88 = 140.0 lbs.

4. Adjust the Minimum Wrestling Weight using the standard error allowance of ± 2% for skinfold measurements (the error may differ depending on the specific methods of skinfold used.)
    132.5 x (1 - 0.02)
    132.5 x 0.98 = 129.9

  <u>Minimum wrestling weight for the season is 129.9 lbs. (130 lb weight class).</u>

5. To Calculate Your Maximum Fat Weight Loss:
  Subtract your calculated minimum body weight from your present weight:
    140 - 129.9 = 10.1 lbs. of fat weight to lose

APPENDX B: Sample Meal Plans

These menus are examples of how to create a balanced meal plan, adapted from The Wrestler's Diet: A Guide to Healthy Weight Control[1]. The snacks provide extra calories and spread out eating throughout the day. **Keep in mind that intensely training athletes need between 2800 to 6000 calories a day and additional hydration (much more than in these examples), depending on individual needs.** Before practice snacks should be eaten between 1½ to 2 hours before practice, and after practice snacks between 15 and 30 minutes after practice.

Calories

Breakfast
Blender Drink

Banana, 1	100
Milk, 1 cup 2%	120
Peanut Butter, 1t	98
Toast, 1 slice	70
Jam, 1t	15
Calories	400

Mid-morning Snack
Pretzels, thin, 10	240
Yogurt, fruit flavored, 8 0z	230
Nectarines, 2	130
Water, 12 oz	0

Lunch
Hamburger on Bun

Bun	120
Ground Beef, 2 oz	120
Catsup, 1T	20
French Fries	220
Milk, 1 cup 2%	120
Oatmeal Raisin Cookies, 2 (2 1/2" diameter)	120
Calories	760

Before Practice Snack
Grape Juice, 1 C	125
Apricots (3)	50

After Practice Snack
Orange Juice, 6 oz	80

Dinner
Roast Pork, 3 oz	220
Baked Potato	100
Broccoli, 1 stalk	20
Margarine, 2t	70
Bread, 1 slice	70
Sliced peaches, 1 cup	130
Milk, 1 cup 2%	120
Calories	730

Evening Snack
Lo-cal Pudding, 1 cup	130

Total Calories	2838

Calories

Breakfast
Grapefruit Juice, 6 oz	75
Unsweetened Cereal, 1 cup	110
Banana, 1 medium	100
Milk, 1 cup 2%	120
Toast, 1 slice	70
Margarine, 1t	35
Jam, 1t	15
Calories	525

Mid-morning Snack
Celery Sticks	10
Peanut Butter, 1t	98
Tomato Juice, 1C	40
Oatmeal Bread, 1 slice	65

Lunch
Chicken Salad Sandwich

Bread, 2 slices	140
Chicken Breast, 2 oz	120
Lo Cal Dressing, 1T	30
Milk, 1 C 2%	120
Apple, 1 medium	80
Calories	490

Before Practice Snack
Popsicle	70
Cheerios®, 1 oz	110

After Practice Snack
Grape Juice, 1 C	125

Dinner
Chili, 2 cups	600
Saltine® Crackers, 12	160
Cheddar Cheese, 2 oz	225
Milk, 1 cup 2%	120
Carrot and Celery Sticks	10
Calories	890

Evening Snack
Orange, 1 medium	80

Total Calories	2728

Calories

Breakfast
Apple Juice, 6 oz................................. 90
Oatmeal, 1 cup.................................... 145
Raisins, 1T... 30
Milk, 1 cup 2%.................................... 120
Toast, 1 slice...................................... 70
Margarine... 35
Calories... 490

Mid-morning Snack
Hard Boiled Eggs, 2........................ 150
Honeydew Melon, 2 slices................ 90

Lunch
Sloppy Joe
  Hamburger Filling, 2 oz..................... 200
  Bun.. 140
Carrot and Celery Sticks......................... 10
Milk, 1 cup 2%.................................... 120
Chocolate Chip Cookie, 1 small............ 50
Calories... 520

Before Practice Snack
Apple, 1 meduim............................ 80
Granola Bar.................................. 110
Grapefuit Juice, 6 oz...................... 75

After Practice Snack
Chocolate Milk, 1 cup 2%.................. 180

Dinner
Turkey Tacos
  Taco Shells, 3................................ 210
  Picante Sauce, 2 oz......................... 30
  American Cheese, 4 oz. shredded........ 220
  Ground Turkey, 4 oz....................... 310
  Lettuce, Onion, Tomato, etc............. 10
Milk, 2 cup 2%................................. 240
Calories... 900

Evening Snack
Orange, 1 medium............................ 80
Provolone Cheese, 1 oz..................... 100

Total Calories..................................... 2895

Calories

Breakfast
Orange Juice 6 oz.............................. 80
English Muffin................................... 140
Peanut Butter, 1T.............................. 90
Banana, 1 medium.............................. 100
Milk, 1 cup 2%.................................. 120
Calories... 530

Mid-morning Snack
Malt-O-Meal®, 1 cup.................. 120
Orange, 1 meduim..................... 80

Lunch
Cheese Pizza, 2 slices........................ 400
Milk, 1 cup 2%.................................. 120
Apple, 1 medium............................... 80
Calories... 600

Before Practice Snack
Granola bar, 2............................. 220
Apricots, 3.................................. 50
Chocolate Milk, 1 cup 2%.................. 180

After Practice Snack
Apple Juice, 6 oz.............................. 90

Dinner
Chicken and Noodles, 1 cup............... 300
Cooked Carrots, 1/2 cup..................... 25
Lettuce Salad................................... 10
Dressing, 1T.................................... 60
Milk, 1 cup 2%.................................. 120
Calories... 515

Evening Snack
Milk, 1 cup 2%................................. 120
Fig Bars, 5...................................... 250

Total Calories................................... 2655

Nicholas Rizzo, M.D.

Breakfast   Calories
French Toast, 2 slices.................................. 300
Syrup, 2 oz... 200
Strawberries, 4 oz., unsweetened................. 25
Milk, 1 cup 2%.. 120
Calories... 645

Mid-morning Snack
Saltine® crackers, 5............................. 63
Margarine, 1 T...................................... 75
Apple Juice, 1 cup................................ 117

Lunch
Turkey Sandwich
  Bread, 2 slices.................................. 140
  Turkey Breast, 3 oz............................ 105
  Lettuce, Tomato Slices........................ 5
  Lo-cal Mayonnaise, 1T........................ 30
Milk, 1 cup 2%...................................... 120
Calories... 400

Before Practice Snack
Cheddar Cheese, 2 oz........................... 225
Apple, 1.. 81
Orange Juice, 1 cup.............................. 110

After Practice Snack
Grapefuit Juice, 6 oz............................ 75

Dinner
Beef Stew, 2 cups................................ 400
Dinner Roll, 1...................................... 70
Margarine, 1t....................................... 35
Applesauce, 4 oz.................................. 55
Milk, 1 cup 2%..................................... 120
Lo-cal Pudding, 1 cup........................... 130
Vanilla Wafers, 6.................................. 100
Calories.. 910

Evening Snack
Popcorn, 2 cups, no Butter..................... 60
Grapes, ½ cup...................................... 100
Diet Soda, 12 oz................................... 0

Total Calories................................. 2861

Breakfast   Calories
Cantaloupe, 1/4..................................... 60
Eggs, poached, 2................................... 150
Toast, 2 slices...................................... 140
Margarine, 1t.. 35
Jam, 2t.. 30
Milk, 1 cup 2%...................................... 120
Calories... 535

Mid-morning Snack
Plain Bagel.. 200
Margarine, 1 T...................................... 75
Jam or Preserves, 1 tsp.......................... 54
Pear, 1... 120
Sports Drink, 16 oz............................... 100

Lunch
Tuna Pocket
  Pita Bread, 1.................................... 120
  Tuna, 3 oz....................................... 100
  Lo-cal Mayonnaise, 2T........................ 60
  Lettuce, Tomato Slices........................ 5
Pretzels, 2 oz....................................... 220
Milk, 1 cup 2%...................................... 120
Calories... 515

Before Practice Snack
Dutch-type Pretzels, 3........................... 187
Grapes, 1 cup...................................... 200
Sports Drink, 16 oz............................... 29

After Practice Snack
Apple Juice, 1 cup................................ 117

Dinner
Broiled Turkey Breast, 3 oz..................... 130
Wild Rice Pilaf, 1 cup............................ 270
Spinach Salad....................................... 15
Dressing, 1T.. 60
Angel Food Cake, 1 slice........................ 125
Chocolate Syrup, 2T.............................. 75
Milk, 2 cup 2%..................................... 240
Calories.. 795

Evening Snack
Pineapple, 1 cup................................... 150
Graham Crackers, 6 squares.................... 160
Orange Juice, 1 cup.............................. 110

Total Calories................................. 3577

APPENDIX C: Sample Restaurant Menus

Adapted from The Wrestler's Diet: A Guide to Healthy Weight Control[1]. <u>NOTE</u>: most of these and other restaurants have their nutritional information on their web sites.

	Calories	Protein	Carbs	Fat
## Breakfast				
McDonald's®				
Plain English Muffin (S)	747	17%	56%	25%
Strawberry jam (1 packet)				
Scrambled egg (1)				
Orange Juice (6 ounces)				
2 % milk (1 carton)				
or Hot Cakes with	650	11%	66%	25%
butter* and 1/2 syrup pack				
orange juice				
*if still hungry order a plain English muffin				
Family Style Restaurant				
Buttermilk Pancakes 5" (3)	761	12%	667%	20%
Butter (a pat)				
Egg (1)				
Syrup (3 tablespoons)				
Orange juice (6 ounces)				
(Usually comes with two eggs. Order one instead. Poached, soft or hard-boiled is recommended.)				
or Cold cereal with	668	15%	58%	26%
2% milk (4 oz.)				
Egg (1)				
English muffin				
Butter (1 pat)				
Jelly (1 packet)				
Orange juice (4oz.)				
## Lunch/Dinner				
McDonald's®				
Chicken Sandwich with	677	22%	53%	25%
BBQ sauce				
Side salad				
1/2 packet low-calorie vinegar and oil dressing				
Orange juice (6 oz.)				
2% milk (1 carton)				
Wendy's®				
Chicken breast Sandwich	719	22%	53%	25%
on multigrain bread				
(no mayonnaise)				
Baked potato				
Sour cream (1 packet)				
2 % milk				
or Chili (8 ounces)	1,016	16%	57%	25%
Baked potato, plain				
Frosty (small)				
Side Salad: 3/4 cup lettuce, 3/4 cup fresh veggies, 1/4 cup cottage cheese				

	Calories	Protein	Carbs	Fat

Lunch/Dinner (continued)

Arby's®

Jr. Roast Beef on
  multigrain bread with lettuce
  and tomato (no mayonnaise or
  horseradish)
Side salad*
2 % milk

695   22%   51%   27%

---

or Arby's Regular Roast
  Beef or ham and cheese sandwich
Side salad*
Vanilla shake
*1/2 cup lettuce, 1 cup fresh veggies, 1/2 cup garbanzo beans, 1/4
  cup cottage cheese, 2 tablespoons low-calorie dressing

970   20%   52%   30%

Taco Bell®

2 tostadas*
1 bean burrito
2 plain tortillas
2% milk

1,040   18%   56%   27%

---

or 1 tostadas*
2 bean burritos
1 plain tortilla
2% milk

1,105   18%   55%   28%

---

or 3 tostadas*
1 plain tortilla
2% milk
*if possible, ask that tostada shell be plain, not fried

785   19%   53%   28%

Pizza Hut®*

Large Spaghetti with
  meat sauce
Breadsticks
2% milk

1,023   19%   61%   20%

---

or 1/2 medium onion,
  green pepper and cheese
  pizza (thin crust)
2 breadsticks
2% milk
*Pizza Hut does have a salad bar.

1,126   20%   55%   25%

Family Style Restaurant

Baked fish
Baked potato with sour cream (1T)
1 muffin
Salad bar (1 cup lettuce)
2% milk (8 oz.)
Sherbet (1/2 cup)

1,100   25%   51%   23%

APPENDIX D: Selected Web Sites

Note: the author is not affiliated/associated with these web sites in any way. Content of web sites may change at any time.

Nutrition & Health

American Dietetic Association	www.ada.org
Anorexia Nervosa and Related Eating Disorders	www.anred.org
Food and Drug Administration	http://vm.cfsan.fda.gov/~dms/foodlab.html

(This page on the FDA's website gives an excellent overview of Food Labels.)

Nutrition in Complementary Care	www.complementarynutrition.org
Olen Publishing, Inc.	www.olen.com/food

(This link gives nutitional information for fast foods based on their book "Fast Food Facts®".)

Scan: Sports, Cardiovascular and Wellness Nutritionists	www.nutrifit.org
Vegetarian Resource Group	www.vrg.org

Wrestling & Sports Fitness

Amatuer Wrestling News	www.amatuerwrestlingnews.com
American College of Sports Medicine	www.acsm.org
The Arsenal: The Wrestler's Training Log	www.arsenaltraining.com
Gatorade Sports Science Institute	www.gssiweb.com
National Athletic Trainers' Association	www.nata.org
The National Collegiate Athletic Association	www.ncaa.org
National Wrestling Coaches Association	www.themat.com
USA Wrestling	www.wrestlingusa.com

Restaurants (These are the restaurants' home pages or nutritional information pages. This list is found on www.NCAA.org.)

Arby's®	www.arbys.com/arb06.html
Baskin-Robbins®	www.baskinrobbins.com/about/nutritional.shtml
Boston Market®	www.bostonmarket.com/2_food/2_2_nutrition/nutrition.htm
Chick-fil-A®	www.chick-fil-a.com
Dairy Queen®	www.dairyqueen.com/menus/men_nutrition.asp
Fazoli's®	www.fazolis.com/nutrition.asp
Hardees®	www.hardeesrestaurants.com/nutrition
White Castle®	www.whitecastle.com/feed/feed_nutrition.html
Kentucky Fried Chicken®	www.kfc.com/food/nutrition.asp
Long John Silver's®	www.ljsilvers.com/nutrition/nutrition.htm
McDonald's®	www.mcdonalds.com/countries/usa/food/nutrition_facts/index.html
Subway®	www.subway.com
Papa John's®	www.papajohns.com/menu/original.htm
Pizza Hut®	www.pizzahut.com/more.asp
Schlotzsky's Deli®	www.cooldeli.com/nutri_original.html
Taco Bell®	www.tacobell.com
Wendy's®	www.wendys.com/w-4-2-25.shtml

APPENDIX E: Carb Reference Chart

Adapted from "The Truth About Carbs: Their Role in Healthy, Long-term Weight Loss", by WeightWatchers International, Inc.[27]

Type of Food	Examples	Type of Carb	Also Provides
Whole Grains	Brown Rice Whole-wheat Pasta 100% Whole-wheat Bread Rolled Oats High-fiber Breakfast Cereal	Concentrated, starchy (complex) carbs, minimally processed	◆ Calories ◆ Essential Nutrients ◆ Fiber ◆ Minerals ◆ Vitamins ◆ Very good eating satisfaction
Whole Vegetables	Lettuce Tomatoes Beans Carrots Corn Baked Potatoes	Less concentrated starchy carb, minimally processed	
Whole Fruits	Peaches Apples Berries Melons	Natural sugars, minimally processed	
Dairy Products	Milk Unsweetened Yogurt		
Refined Grains	Traditional Breads, Cereals and Pastas made from Processed Flour White Rice	Concentrated starchy carbs, processed in a form that removes some nutrients	◆ Calories ◆ Some Nutrients (kept or added back after processing) ◆ Convenience
Fruit Juices and Vegetable Juices	100% Orange Juice Tomato Juice	Concentrated source of natural sugars	
Convenience and Packaged Foods	Boxed Dinner Entrées Spaghetti Sauce and other Cooking Sauces	Refined grains and/or highly processed foods, lots of added sugars and starch	
Sweets and Snack Foods*	Cookies Cakes Ice Cream Candy	Very concentrated source of added, processed sugars	◆ A lot of calories without essential nutrients ◆ Eating pleasure by indulgence or satisfying a craving
Spreads and Condiments	Jellies and Jams Table Sugar Honey		
Beverages	Fruit-flavored Drinks Soda Pop		

*These usually contain a lot of added, processed fat in addition to sugars, making them an even more concentrated source of empty calories.

BONUS SECTION: Handouts on Skin Care and Common Injuries

<u>Note</u>: The health and instructional disclaimer at the beginning of this book also applies to each of these handouts.

The following pages are designed to be copied and distributed to wrestlers, their parents and coaches. *The following pages only* are free from the copyright restrictions on the rest of this book:

WRESTLING HANDOUT #1: Cauliflower Ear
WRESTLING HANDOUT #2: Concussions
WRESTLING HANDOUT #3: Head Injury Fact Sheet
WRESTLING HANDOUT #4: Guidelines for Parents of Children in Sports
WRESTLING HANDOUT #5: Herpes & Cold Sores
WRESTLING HANDOUT #6: Illness Prevention
WRESTLING HANDOUT #7: Impetigo
WRESTLING HANDOUT #8: Muscle Cramps
WRESTLING HANDOUT #9: Nosebleeds
WRESTLING HANDOUT #10: Ringworm
WRESTLING HANDOUT #11: Rules of the Room
WRESTLING HANDOUT #12: Skin Care
WRESTLING HANDOUT #13: Strains & Sprains
WRESTLING HANDOUT #14: When to Use Heat and Cold for Injuries

WRESTLING HANDOUT #1: Cauliflower Ear

Athletes involved in any contact sport can suffer a contusion to the ear which may result in a "cauliflower" ear (also called auricular hematoma). It is a deformity of the outer ear most commonly seen in wrestling, rugby, boxing, football and judo. It occurs after someone gets a blow or repeated blows to the ear, enough for a large blood clot (lump of blood) to develop under the skin or for the ear's skin to be stripped away from the cartilage (the flexible material that gives the ear its shape). The body normally absorbs excess fluid or blood at an injury site over time, but not always in the ear because of its special structure. The cartilage of the ear has no blood supply except that supplied by the ear's skin. When the the cartilage receives little or no blood flow because of tearing of the skin, bruising or a blood clot, it eventually dies and is replaced by scar tissue. An acute cauliflower ear is often painful and causes swelling. If left untreated, it results in deformation of the ear which may last for life.

Unfortunately, most wrestlers do not seek care until the bleeding and swelling have stabilized and resulted in deformity. By not getting medical care immediately, they increase their risk of infection, recurrence, scarring and deformity. After a cauliflower ear has formed and hardened, it will not recover its normal shape without surgery. But if caught and treated early enough, a person usually will not get a significant lifelong deformity.

High school and college wrestling rules require the use of protective headgear, but problems still occur. Not wearing headgear or wearing poorly fitting headgear is a big factor in causing cauliflower ear. (Freestyle and Greco-Roman do not require headgear for juniors and prohibit use on the international level.)

Treatment

At first, the swelling will be soft and mushy fluid. It is at this early stage that immediate treatment can help decrease or avoid permanent scarring. If the fluid is allowed to solidify, it will cause permanent disfiguration.

Immediate care should include ice and a head wrap (elastic gauze with packing material in front and behind ear, applying moderate pressure). This wrapping should not cause a headache, block vision, or cover the other ear. After that, the next step is one of the following: drainage (aspiration) and compression, drainage and splinting with various materials, or incision and drainage with clot removal. Sometimes stitches are needed if there is a tear in the skin. Your doctor may prescribe antibiotics to prevent an infection.

Drainage and Compression: A doctor can drain the blood from the ear either with a syringe or through a cut and then help the skin reconnect to the cartilage by applying pressure with a tight bandage.

Drainage and Splinting: Splinting is a medical procedure that keeps pressure on the area of hematoma formation. Sometimes sutures through the ear keep special gauze in place, or sometimes special materials (pediplast or silicone) are molded to the ear. After a splint is placed, the ear should be rechecked by your doctor in seven days. Sutures typically stay in for 14 days, but may be removed if redness or tenderness occurs. The risk of recurrence decreases the longer the splint stays in place. You may to return to wrestling 24 hours after a splint is applied.

<u>Incision and Drainage with Clot Removal</u>: This is a surgical procedure for more serious cauliflower ears, and should only be done by an Ear, Nose and Throat surgeon (also called an ENT or otolaryngologist) or a plastic surgeon.

The best protection from recurrence is to wear properly fitting headgear. Recurrence should be managed immediately and aggressively, with either aspiration and resplinting for one more week or referral to a surgeon for incision, drainage and resplinting. *Severe infections can occur in cauliflower ears and should be treated immediately with open drainage by a surgeon and intravenous antibiotics.*

DO:
- Apply direct pressure with a sterile gauze sponge. Apply pressure by simply pinching the site. Keep the pressure on for at least six minutes.
- Keep the ear dry for 24 hours and apply antibacterial ointment (like Bacitracin® or Neosporin®) twice a day.
- Wait 24 hours before returning to the mats.
- Wrap must remain in place for at least 24 hours. Tape any ear splints from the doctor in the ear during practice.
- Ice the ear a few times each day for 10 to 15 minutes at a time (and especially after practice) for three weeks. Be sure there is a towel between the ice and the ear to avoid frostbite. When icing the ear it should not be dark in color or be painful.
- Make a donut-shaped pad from athletic foam or plastizote and tape it to the inside of the headgear (athletic foam is usually available from the trainers). *Use this for the rest of the season.* Headgear must be properly fitted to your head, so have your coach check both the foam pad and the fit of your headgear.
- Use duct tape for head wrap to apply pressure during practice. (It is better than athletic tape because it stays sticky even with sweat.)
- When wrapping the ear, leave the uninvolved ear exposed.

DON'T:
- Don't pick or press on the ear.
- Don't use loose or poorly-fitting headgear.
- Don't delay getting treatment thinking it will keep you from returning to the mats.

CALL YOUR DOCTOR IF:
- You develop a headache or fever.
- You develop any redness, tenderness, pus drainage, swelling or increased pain.
- You have any change in hearing.

References: 1. "Management of Wrestler's Cauliflower Ear", HealthSouth of Southern Nevada, www.geocities.com/hsathletictraining, 2002
2. Sandra E. Lane, MD; Gary L. Rhame, DO; Randall L. Wroble, MD, "A Silicone Splint for Auricular Hematoma", *The Physician and Sportsmedicine*, 26(9), September 1998

From *"Championship Nutrition and Performance: The Wrestler's Guide to Lifestyle, Diet and Healthy Weight Control"* by N. Rizzo, M.D., available at **www.wrestlerdiet.com**.

WRESTLING HANDOUT #2: Concussions*

A Word About Head Injuries

While most head injuries are minor with no long-term consequences, they can damage the scalp, skull, brain or eyes (or a combination of these), and can vary in severity from minor to life threatening. Do not judge the severity of a head injury by its appearance because serious brain or other damage can occur with no sign of damage to the head. For example, if the head is struck, the brain can be bruised as it moves violently within the skull. The brain may also be damaged by pressure inside the skull due to a buildup of fluid or bleeding in the brain after the injury. Initial symptoms often develop soon afterward and, in minor cases, commonly include a mild headache and a lump, bruise or cut on the scalp. Most athletes with a minor head injury recover completely within a few days. However, sometimes an injured person appears well at first and then symptoms of a more serious head injury develop hours or days later. Though CT scans and other medical tests may show abnormalities with head injuries, they may not always show problems associated with the mild head injuries typical in athletic competition. The outcome of a serious head injury is often difficult to predict. Recovery may take up to two years and problems such as speech problems, coma, paralysis and death may occur. Concussions are one type of head injury.

Concussions

A concussion is an injury to the brain caused by a blow to the head or by striking the head on something. This causes a mild abnormality in normal brain function. The initial symptoms of a concussion are similar to that of more serious head injuries like bleeding into the brain. The difference is that symptoms of a concussion should show steady improvement over a short period after the initial injury. If symptoms are worsening or not improving, there is cause to worry about swelling or bleeding inside the skull. The signs and symptoms of a concussion include temporary loss of consciousness, confusion, loss of memory about the event that related to the concussion as well as some time before or after (amnesia), dizziness, headache, mild lack of coordination, nausea and vomiting, and inability to concentrate. These symptoms usually get better in a few hours or days.

Second Impact Syndrome and Post-concussional Syndrome

Second-impact syndrome is a rapid, deadly brain swelling that may occur if a person who has had a concussion suffers another head impact -- even a minor one -- before the symptoms of a previous concussion have fully cleared. Even after recovery, an athlete's chance of suffering another concussion may be four times as high as that of someone who has never had a concussion. And repeated concussions could cause permanent brain damage or death. This is the reason for the strict return-to-play guidelines for concussions. However, the risk of getting second-impact syndrome does diminish with time.

Following a concussion, a few people develop post-concussional syndrome -- a collection of symptoms that may follow a concussion. These include headache, poor concentration, mild memory loss, irritability, trouble sleeping, nightmares and sometimes mild personality or behavior changes. Treatment consists of watchful waiting until the symptoms resolve. There are no treatments or medicines that will shorten the recovery time. It goes away on its own and you should gradually improve to their normal pre-injury state.

Although this condition may last from weeks to months, it is important to remember that it will get better. If you are diagnosed with post-concussional syndrome, avoid making life-changing decisions such as quitting school or changing jobs because of the symptoms that you are experiencing. Changing some things at work or school environments may help minimize the problems of any memory loss or difficulties in concentration. Support from friends and family may help you remember that this is a temporary condition.

Treatment

Your doctor will examine you and, if necessary, may order tests at the hospital like X-rays to look for a fracture and MRI or CT scanning to look for swelling or bleeding. Your doctor may admit you to the hospital for observation overnight. The main treatment is rest and careful observation. If your doctor does not admit you to the hospital you can be safely observed at home by a family member or close friend -- they may notice changes in normal behavior that a medical person who does not know you might miss. If you have a severe headache, a cut that requires stitches, a loss of consciousness (even if brief), if you are concerned about the severity of the injury, or if additional symptoms develop you must go to the hospital or get medical help at once. Many individuals will have a headache and physical activity may make it worse. If you did not lose consciousness at the time of the concussion and have only a mild headache, it is safe to take Tylenol® (acetaminophen) to relieve the pain. You probably do not need to be at bed rest, but you should keep your activity light and get plenty of rest until you are feeling normal. An ice pack to the area struck by the original blow may help with pain for the first few days. You should take all precautions to avoid another concussion in the near future.

Return to Play Guidelines

Return-to-play guidelines attempt to decrease the risks of further injury and second-impact syndrome by taking into account injury severity and not allowing you to return to competition if symptoms are present. If you still have symptoms or signs of a concussion, or if exercise alone reproduces symptoms, return to competition is not allowed. But once the symptoms have cleared, there is debate among experts as to how long you should be kept from contact play. As a second concussion (especially within three months of the first one) may result in permanent brain damage and even death, some guidelines recommend that you not do contact sports for three months. Other guidelines suggest anywhere from 20 minutes, a week, a season, or forever depending on the severity of concussion and your personal history. Another example: an athlete who loses consciousness for 30 seconds would have a severe concussion and would be barred from play for one week to a month. Your own feeling regarding return to competition also needs to be considered – if you do not feel ready to return to competition, then you are not ready. **Bottom line: get your doctor's permission and medical clearance *in writing* as to when you may or may not return to competition. Be sure that your parents, coach and trainer have a copy of this written medical clearance.**

*Please also refer to WRESTLING HANDOUT #3: Head Injury Fact Sheet.

From "*Championship Nutrition and Performance: The Wrestler's Guide to Lifestyle, Diet and Healthy Weight Control*" by N. Rizzo, M.D., available at **www.wrestlerdiet.com**.

WRESTLING HANDOUT #3: Head Injury Fact Sheet*

Often, signs of a head injury do not appear immediately after trauma, but hours and even days after an injury. The purpose of this fact sheet is to alert you to the symptoms of head injuries that may occur several hours afterward, point out the seriousness of these symptoms and that they require immediate medical help, and instruct you in the proper care of head injury symptoms.

WATCH FOR THE FOLLOWING SIGNS AND SYMPTOMS THAT MAY INDICATE A SERIOUS HEAD INJURY WITH INCREASING PRESSURE FROM BRAIN SWELLING AND/OR BLEEDING. IF YOU GET ANY OF THE FOLLOWING SIGNS OR SYMPTOMS TALK TO YOUR DOCTOR AND ACTIVATE THE EMERGENCY MEDICAL SYSTEM (CALL 911) OR GO TO THE EMERGENCY ROOM IMMEDIATELY.

- Continuing or worsening headache
- Loss of appetite, nausea or vomiting
- Abnormal or increased drowsiness, unusual sleepiness, or difficulty awakening
- Uncontrollable shaking, jerking or convulsions (seizures)
- Blood or clear fluid coming from the ears or nose
- Slurred or garbled speech, or any other changes in speaking
- Slowing heart rate
- Ringing in the ears
- Stiff neck
- Blurred or double vision, one pupil larger than the other, abnormal eye movements or shaking eyes
- Increasing or persistent confusion or problems with memory (like difficulty remembering recent events or important facts)
- Unusual sensations like tingling or numbness of the arms, hands or fingers
- Behavior changes (irritability, restlessness, crying, excessive laughter, obnoxious behavior, moodiness)
- Clumsiness, weakness or loss of strength in arms or legs (on either or both sides), difficulty walking, dizziness, staggering, poor balance or unsteadiness
- If you have any worsening of symptoms, if you are not improved within about 24 hours, or have any other signs or symptoms that concern you

Follow these "DO's" and "DON'T's"

DO:

- It is important that you are not alone and a responsible family member or friend is with you for the next 24 to 72 hours, or longer until you are feeling back to normal. Give him/her this sheet and your doctor's name and phone number. Have them wake you every 2 to 3 hours the first 24 hours.
- Many people with concussions have nausea, so eat a light diet for the first 24 to 48 hours. A heavy diet may lead to vomiting. Begin with clear liquids and advance to solids as tolerated.
- Return to activity only after your doctor has given you full medical clearance *in writing*. Give a copy of this written clearance to your parents and coach/trainer.

DON'T:

- ♦ Don't take any medicines or substances that cause drowsiness or changes in levels of consciousness including narcotic pain medicines, alcohol, sleeping pills, muscle relaxants, antihistamines (allergy pills), tranquilizers or recreational drugs.
- ♦ Don't take any medications without first calling the doctor. Do **NOT** take aspirin or other anti-inflammatory medicines like ibuprofen for the first 24 hours as they may make bleeding worse. If you did not lose consciousness and have only a mild headache, you may take Tylenol® (acetaminophen).
- ♦ Don't take medicines such as stimulants or decongestants because they may aggravate irritability.
- ♦ Don't drive. Don't do any sports (including swimming and hunting). Don't take a tub bath. Don't operate dangerous or heavy machinery.
- ♦ Don't do strenuous activities until cleared by your doctor. This may result in a more severe headache.
- ♦ Don't do activities that may result in another concussion.
- ♦ Limit physical activity for 24 hours. No school for students, no work for adults.

If Someone Loses Consciousness or Has a Seizure:

1. Instruct someone to call 911 or your emergency number immediately to get help.
2. If they are standing, try to prevent or break the fall.
3. Turn the person onto one side.
4. Loosen any tight clothing around the neck. If there is the possibility of a head or neck injury and if the airway is clear, do not remove the headgear – leave that to the emergency personnel.
5. Remove any object in the immediate area that could cause injury (such as hard or sharp objects).
6. Do not put anything in the person's mouth, including your fingers.
7. Let the person lie on one side until the seizure is over. Explain what happened to them and where he or she is.
8. The person may be groggy and confused afterwards if he/she regains consciousness. Stay with the person and instruct them to lie still until help arrives.

For More Information: Brain Injury Association, www.biausa.org

EMERGENCY CONTACT PHONE NUMBERS:

Parents/Guardian: _____   **Doctor:** _____

Emergency Medical: _____   **Coach:** _____

*Also refer to WRESTLING HANDOUT #2: Concussions.

From *"Championship Nutrition and Performance: The Wrestler's Guide to Lifestyle, Diet and Healthy Weight Control"* by N. Rizzo, M.D., available at **www.wrestlerdiet.com**.

WRESTLING HANDOUT #4: Guidelines for Parents of Children in Sports*

1. Make sure your children know that – win or lose – you love them and are not disappointed with their performance.

2. Be realistic about your child's physical ability.

3. Help your child set realistic goals.

4. Emphasize improved performance, not winning. Positively reinforce improved skills.

5. Do not relive your own athletic past through your child.

6. Provide a safe environment for training and competition. This includes proper training methods, proper use of equipment, proper nutrition, and getting proper medical care when needed.

7. Control your own negative emotions at meets and tournaments. Do not yell at other wrestlers, coaches or officials – it only takes away from your job as a positive role model.

8. Be a cheerleader for your child and the other children on the team.

9. Respect your child's coaches. Be the best parent you can be and let the coaches be the best coaches they can be by letting them do the coaching. If you disagree with their approach, *discuss it with them.* Communicate openly with them.

10. Be a positive role model. Enjoy sports yourself. Set your own goals. Live a healthy lifestyle, including your own stress management, diet and nutrition.

*Adapted from "Guidelines for Parents of Children in Sports", *The Physician and Sportsmedicine*, 16(4):71, 1988.

From *"Championship Nutrition and Performance: The Wrestler's Guide to Lifestyle, Diet and Healthy Weight Control"* by N. Rizzo, M.D., available at **www.wrestlerdiet.com**.

WRESTLING HANDOUT #5: Herpes & Cold Sores

Herpes simplex is a virus in the family of viruses that cause chickenpox, shingles, cold sores and mono (mononucleosis). The main cause is the herpes simplex virus type I, and less often herpes type II. These viruses are the cause of cold sores (also called fever blisters). The initial infections usually happen in childhood. It is estimated that about 80% of all adults have had exposure to the virus, but only a few can remember their first infection.

Herpes is mainly transmitted by non-sexual intimate contact with saliva of an infected person; for example, a child kissed by an adult relative whose skin is shedding the virus but who does not yet show signs of an infection. The virus can enter your body through a break in your skin or though the tender skin of your mouth. It is extremely difficult to trace where a person got it because a current outbreak may be the result of an infection acquired months or years ago.

Herpes is usually diagnosed by inspection of the infected site. You may know when a recurrence is about to happen because you may feel itching, tingling or pain in the places where you were first infected, then small blisters emerge and go on to form ulcers and crusts. Healing occurs over ten to 14 days. In some circumstances, specific laboratory tests can be used to verify the identity of the virus, but are not usually necessary. This is a chronic infection that is impossible to eradicate, but millions of individuals are living a normal life with the disease. Herpes virus infections are not curable and may recur throughout life.

> **Wrestlers cannot wrestle in practice or competition with herpes infections, fever blisters, or cold sores.**

Treatment

While there is no cure for herpes, the drugs acyclovir, Valtrex® (valacyclovir), and Famvir® (famciclovir) can be very helpful. The treatment for primary episodes is ten days of antiviral medications taken by mouth (but some experts would not treat cold sores). The oral medications speed up healing, can lessen the pain of infections for many people, and can also be used to lessen the number of recurrences. Because herpes can recur with little warning and the virus can be shed from the skin even without lesions, season-long suppression with oral medications is sometimes done, but it is not an FDA-approved indication. If you get more than one or two episodes of herpes during a season, talk to your doctor about this preventative treatment (called prophylaxis). To soothe pain take Tylenol® (acetaminophen), or Motrin® (ibuprofen). Denavir® (penciclovir) is an effective topical cream for treatment of cold sores, but should not be used in place of oral medications for wrestlers with facial herpes. Other topical creams and popular remedies are available (including moisturizing or anesthetic lip balms), but they have not been shown to be of much help. Common side effects of the antiviral medications include nausea, vomiting, and itching. Allergic reactions and side effects of the medication are possible.

DO:

- Definitely see your doctor to be sure of the diagnosis and treatment, and then getting written medical clearance when completely healed.
- Take medication as prescribed by your doctor.
- Avoid stress. Reactivation of the virus can occur with emotional or physical stress and menstruation. Therefore, stress reduction measures such as avoiding stressful situations or learning how to deal with them effectively are important.
- Use sunscreen. Sunlight (UV light) is also a recurrence trigger, and application of sunscreen may help. Apply a sunscreen-containing lip balm before going outdoors and reapply it often. Definitely avoid tanning beds and bright sunlight.
- Learn to recognize the early symptoms of tingling or itching; then avoid close contact with anyone until the sores have completely healed.
- Wash your hands often.
- Keep the lesions clean and dry.
- Talk to your doctor about using medications like acyclovir preventatively if you have more than one or two episodes during the wrestling season.

DON'T:

- Don't wrestle or work out in the wrestling room for at least one full week of treatment with orally taken prescription medication and you are cleared by your trainer or physician.
- Don't share personal items like headgear, wrestling shoes, razors, combs, brushes, hats, soaps, towels, clothing or bedding.
- Don't shave the affected area.
- Do not scratch. Scratching can lead to a secondary bacterial infection.

Never use bleach, peroxide, iodine or other chemical disinfectants. These will not cure it, may scar and may irritate the skin. This may make it look worse to the referee or doctor and delay your return to competition.

CALL YOUR DOCTOR IF:

- You have infections more than four times a year, or more than once or twice during the wrestling season.
- An infection involves a sensitive organ or tissue such as the eye.
- You see or feel any signs or symptoms of recurrence.

For More Information:
American Social Health Association: National Herpes Resource Center, www.ashastd.org/hrc/educate.html

From **"Championship Nutrition and Performance: The Wrestler's Guide to Lifestyle, Diet and Healthy Weight Control"** by N. Rizzo, M.D., available at **www.wrestlerdiet.com**.

WRESTLING HANDOUT #6: Illness Prevention

Prevention of Systemic Illnesses:

Diseases spread by airborne droplet spread (like viral infections such as colds and flu), person-to-person contact or by exposure to common sources of infection (like food poisoning). Neglecting general hygiene practices is often the major factor in the spread of infectious illnesses. Proper hygiene tips to help prevent an illness from spreading through a team are listed under "**DO**" and "**DON'T**" below.

Immunization is an important part of prevention. Flu shots (influenza vaccines) for athletes who compete during the flu season are good for limiting spread through a team, decreasing symptoms in a sick person, and avoiding interruptions in practice and competition. Other vaccinations to consider include Tetanus, Hepatitis A, Hepatitis B, Meningitis (meningococcal), Measles/Mumps/Rubella (MMR) and Chicken Pox (Varicella). Fortunately, most school programs require most of these for entry. Athletes traveling to foreign countries should talk to their doctor to determine which vaccinations they may need such as yellow fever, typhoid fever, cholera, Japanese encephalitis and rabies. Vaccines may result in side effects or allergic reactions.

Fatigue, overtraining and improper nutrition are also risk factors for infection. Get enough rest and sleep. Workouts should be spaced out enough to provide good recovery time, and types of workout activities should be varied to maintain interest and focus. Minimize or handle life stress appropriately.

When You Should and Shouldn't Exercise if Sick:

Whether you can or cannot work out is determined mainly by how sick you are. But, for example, if you have a systemic illness (like the flu, food poisoning or diarrhea) you should not work out at all. But if you have a mild cold you can do workouts like running or lifting weights at home. Strenuous workouts should be avoided. Like many contact sports, wrestling uses two different types of workouts – workouts with contact with other participants and workouts without contact. **If you are contagious, you should not work out with partners from your team or work out in the wrestling room.**

A "neck check" may help you decide if you should work out. You can exercise when sick if your symptoms are all above the neck (like stuffiness, mild sore throat, itchy eyes) and if your symptoms do not worsen with exercise. Try a reduced workout first. If symptoms are tolerable or improve during exercise, gradually increase the intensity. But if your symptoms are severe, below the neck, or generalized (like fever, muscle aches, productive cough, vomiting or diarrhea) it may mean more serious illness and you should rest. If you are this sick, stay home and do not practice or compete until your symptoms have resolved completely. Having one wrestler miss practice is better than having the whole team miss a competition.

DO:

- Wash hands frequently with soap and water, especially before you eat and after you go to the bathroom.

- Minimize contact with people who are obviously sick, including teammates. If you know that a cold or flu is spreading in your community you should avoid crowds, unnecessary travel and close contact with young children. Avoid touching common surfaces in public places, such as countertops or doorknobs.

- Use insect repellents in areas where insect-borne disease like Lyme disease or West Nile Virus are risks.

- Protect ice sources like ice buckets and ice machines to avoid contamination. Allow access to ice chests only by designated personnel like trainers. Ice scoops should be frequently sanitized. Do not put your hands in the ice.

- Keep your own name-labeled water bottle for your use only.

- Get enough rest and sleep.

- Eat a well-balanced diet (with the right amounts of calories, carbs, protein and fats) and stay properly hydrated.

DON'T:

- Don't share water bottles, sports drinks or soda cans.

- Don't share personal items, such as toothbrushes, mouth guards or cosmetics.

- Don't work out if you are badly fatigued, too tired or too ill.

From *"Championship Nutrition and Performance: The Wrestler's Guide to Lifestyle, Diet and Healthy Weight Control"* by N. Rizzo, M.D., available at **www.wrestlerdiet.com**.

WRESTLING HANDOUT #7: Impetigo

Impetigo is a common and mild skin infection seen most often in children and frequently spread among family members. It is caused by common skin bacteria, usually staph (staphylococci) or strep (streptococci). It is very contagious and is spread by person to person contact. Risk of getting impetigo increases with poor nutrition, illness (which lowers the body's resistance), warm, and moist enviroments (like wreslting and weight rooms), and poor hygiene.

Impetigo usually starts as small red bumps or blisters. These can get quite large. A "honey-crusted" drainage is common. If left untreated, impetigo can continue for weeks. Rarely, kidney inflammation occurs after impetigo, causing blood or protein in the urine.

> **Wrestlers cannot wrestle in practice or competition with impetigo.**

Treatment

Impetigo is curable with antibiotic creams or with medication taken by mouth. You can expect improvement in five to ten days. Bactroban® is one antibiotic ointment used. Wash the affected area and gently scrub off crusting and loose dead skin with a cloth. Dry off and apply a small amount of Bactroban®. Do this three times a day (about every eight hours). If you are given an antibiotic by mouth, take the entire prescription as directed by your doctor.

DO:

- See your doctor to make the diagnosis, get treatment and obtain medical clearance.
- Maintain good hygiene. Wear clean clothes every day. Shower and shampoo at least once a day. Wash your entire body with an antibacterial soap.
- Launder bedding, clothing and towels frequently.
- Trim finger nails if scratching is a problem.

DON'T:

- Don't wrestle or work out in the wrestling room until 1) at least five full days of treatment, 2) the area looks normal and healed, and 3) you are cleared by your trainer or physician.
- Don't share personal items like headgear, wrestling shoes, razors, combs, brushes, hats, soaps or shampoos, towels, clothing or bedding.
- Don't use over-the-counter medications – they are usually not helpful.
- Don't shave infected areas. If you have to shave use an electric razor.
- Don't break any blisters and avoid scratching.

> **Never use bleach, peroxide, iodine or other chemical disinfectants. These may not cure it, may scar and may irritate the skin. This may make it look worse to the referee or doctor and delay your return to competition.**

CALL YOUR DOCTOR IF:

- You are not better in seven to 10 days.
- You have a temperature of 101° F.
- Other family members become infected.
- Your urine is discolored or there is blood in the urine.

From *"Championship Nutrition and Performance: The Wrestler's Guide to Lifestyle, Diet and Healthy Weight Control"* by N. Rizzo, M.D., available at **www.wrestlerdiet.com**.

WRESTLING HANDOUT #8: Muscle Cramps

Cramps are painful, spasmodic, involuntary contractions of skeletal muscle that occur during or immediately after exercise. Athletes usually get cramping at or near the end of a bout of intense or prolonged exercise, and have distress and pain, a hard contracted muscle, and visible twitching over the muscle belly. If bad enough, muscle cramps can finish an athlete from competition for the day. The muscles most prone to cramping are those that span two joints. Important risk factors include muscle fatigue, shorter daily stretching time, irregular stretching habits, older age, longer history of exercise, and sweating early, heavily and caking with salt.

Although there are many causes of muscle cramps, muscle fatigue, salt loss (sodium loss), and dehydration all play a role in muscle cramping. Sodium is important not only to maintain blood volume but also to help nerves fire and muscles work, so a lack of sodium and fluid may make muscles "irritable". A lack of sodium short-circuits the nerves and muscles as muscles contract and relax. The result can be muscle cramping. Under such conditions, a stress such as movement may cause the muscle to contract and twitch uncontrollably. (The amounts of potassium, calcium and magnesium lost in sweat are low compared to the amounts of sodium and chloride. Potassium, magnesium and calcium are easily replaced by the diet, so a lack of these is rare.) There are some reports that certain dietary supplements such as creatine might increase the risk of muscle cramps. If cramps suddenly occur without a prior history, see a doctor to rule out more serious causes like diabetes, nerve diseases, metabolic diseases or circulation problems.

Prevention

Prevention of cramps is best done by protecting the muscle from developing early fatigue and by doing the following:

- A balanced diet containing some salty foods and proper hydration is the best prevention. Some foods rich in sodium include tomato juice, canned baked beans, dill pickles, pretzels, canned soups and cheese pizza.

- Be in good condition before the wrestling season starts.

- Stretch and warm up properly before competition and workouts.

Treatment

When cramps strike during a workout or competition, take immediate action with stretching, massage and recovery. Because cramps are often related to heavy exercise, stretching and non-weight-bearing movement often help. Rubbing the area may help decrease pain and increase blood flow. Get rest and re-hydration with fluids containing electrolytes, especially sodium. It may be necessary to reduce the exercise intensity and duration. Sometimes the application of heat helps. (See WRESTLING HANDOUT # 14: When to Use Heat & Cold for Athletic Injuries.)

After checking with a doctor to rule out serious causes, wrestlers who get severe muscle cramps or who are "salty sweaters" might want to add some salt to meals. Try adding ¼ teaspoon of salt to a 16 to 20 ounce beverage or by adding an extra shake of the salt shaker at lunch. Salty snacks or an extra tap of the salt shaker will help. Remember, a simple shake of the salt shaker has a lot of sodium in it! Drinking certain sports drinks is also a good way to replace sodium. Athletes should not use salt tablets, unless specifically directed by their trainer or doctor.

DO:

♦ Drink plenty of fluids to stay hydrated throughout the day and during exercise.

♦ Get good nutritional recovery (particularly for salt).

♦ Rest your muscles after hard training.

♦ Passively stretch the affected muscle groups: start by holding the muscle in a stretched position until spasm stops and a return to normal muscle length does not cause a cramp.

♦ Stay at a comfortable temperature.

♦ Go to the medical care facility at the sports event if cramps are severe.

DON'T:

♦ Don't take nutritional or dietary supplements.

♦ Don't use super-salty sources like pickle juice, mustard or antacids as quick "fixes". *These are not proven to work and they usually provide too much salt and not enough fluid.*

CALL YOUR DOCTOR IF:

♦ You experience recurrent acute muscle cramps.

♦ You do not pass any urine or pass very dark urine in the first 24 hours after the cramping.

♦ You have generalized severe cramping (in non-exercising muscle groups) or have localized cramping accompanied by confusion, sleepiness, coma or other problems. These may be signs of a serious medical condition that may require immediate hospitalization.

From *"Championship Nutrition and Performance: The Wrestler's Guide to Lifestyle, Diet and Healthy Weight Control"* by N. Rizzo, M.D., available at **www.wrestlerdiet.com**.

WRESTLING HANDOUT #9: Nosebleeds

Nosebleeds (also called epistaxis) are often caused by injuring the membranes of a blood vessel in the nose with cotton swabs, finger tips, hard nose-blowing, objects falling on the nose or other trauma. Other causes include chemical irritants, infections, or abnormalities of the blood vessels of the nose. Diseases, such as high blood pressure or blood clotting disorders, may also cause a nosebleed. The most common cause is excessive drying of the nasal passages from dry air, especially in the winter. They are twice as common in children. Most resolve with direct pressure on the nose, although some may need further medical intervention such as packing or cautery.

The nose may bleed from one or both nostrils. There also may be bleeding down the back of the throat with spitting of blood, coughing of blood, or vomiting of blood. Swallowed blood irritates the stomach frequently causing vomiting. Most nosebleeds do not result in enough blood loss to cause problems. But, a very prolonged, heavy nosebleed may result in a low blood level (anemia). If you have had a large nosebleed recently, you may notice dark or tar-like bowel movements – these are a sign that you have swallowed a significant amount of blood. (The dark color is from digested blood.)

Treatment

The first-line treatment is direct pressure. If this is not successful during a match, a trainer or team doctor may pack the nose with cotton or apply certain medicines to stop the bleeding. Grasp the nose firmly between the thumb and first finger and squeeze it for ten to 30 minutes without releasing the nose or peeking. Placing an ice pack on the bridge of the nose may help slow the blood flow to the nose. Lean your head slightly forward (tuck your chin into your chest) so that any blood running down the throat may be spit out rather than swallowed. This may help prevent vomiting.

If you continue to bleed, it may be necessary to have the nose treated by a doctor. Your doctor may do one or more of the following: pack absorbent gauze into the nose so as to place pressure on the bleeding site, apply medicines to the bleeding areas to help stop the bleeding, or cauterize bleeding blood vessels. The main side effects of packing are discomfort, an inability to breathe through your nose, and an increased risk of sinus infection. (In some people, there is also a risk of slowed heart rate or decreased blood pressure, and the doctor may recommend hopitalization.)

DO:

♦ Remain in a sitting position with your head slightly forward (chin to chest) and squeeze the lower half of your nose with your thumb and index finger for ten to 30 minutes.

♦ Keep your mouth open if you have to sneeze.

♦ If the nosebleed is caused by high blood pressure, work with your doctor to get your blood pressure under good control.

♦ Humidify the air in your home and, if possible, at work.

- On the second day, place a little petroleum jelly just inside your nostril to protect it from drying and to soften any crusts that form.

- A scarf or cloth mask may be helpful if you have to be out in cold, dry air.

- Use over-the-counter saline (salt water) nasal sprays if dryness is a problem.

- If irritating chemicals or dusts are a problem, avoid them or use a filter-type mask.

- If you had packing put in by a doctor, make an appointment with that doctor to have it removed. *Do no remove medical packing yourself!*

DON'T:

- Don't blow your nose forcefully or blow out any clots.

- Don't pick your nose, pick at any clots, or put anything into it (cotton swabs, handkerchief corners, tissue).

- If you get nosebleeds often, avoid things that cause them like dry air.

- Don't use decongestant nasal sprays – they can be a problem, and you should discuss them with your doctor.

- Avoid coffee, tea, or alcohol until at least 24 hours after bleeding has stopped.

- Don't bend, stoop, lift or do strenuous exercise.

- Don't take aspirin, ibuprofen or other anti-inflammatory medications because they may slow clotting and promote bleeding.

CALL YOUR DOCTOR IF:

- Your nose is gushing.

- You vomit from swallowed blood.

- If you are still bleeding after 30 minutes of pressure.

- You are having more than three or four nosebleeds a day.

- You have a temperature of greater than 102° F, especially if your nose was packed or cauterized.

- If you have a new or persistent headache.

- If allergies or infections are a problem.

- Your nosebleeds are caused by high blood pressure or a blood problem or a bleeding disease like anemia, hemophilia or leukemia.

- You are taking antiinflammatories like aspirin or ibuprofen, or are on blood thinners like as heparin or warfarin.

From *"Championship Nutrition and Performance: The Wrestler's Guide to Lifestyle, Diet and Healthy Weight Control"* by N. Rizzo, M.D., available at **www.wrestlerdiet.com**.

WRESTLING HANDOUT #10: Ringworm & Tinea

Ringworm and Tinea are general terms used to describe common and very contagious skin infections. They are not caused by a "worm" but by a fungus. Fungi are found everywhere and are extremely small, being seen only with a microscope. Ringworm and tinea are transmitted from other individuals or animals, or by contact with infected surfaces such as towels, carpet, bedding, weight rooms, tanning beds, showers and baths. Ringworm is much more common in hot, humid weather and can occur at any age. Risk of getting it increases with crowded living conditions, daycare centers or schools, decreased resistance to infection caused by illnesses or drugs, chronic moisture, and chafing of the skin. The diagnosis of ringworm can usually be made by its typical appearance on the skin. In unusual cases, a small scraping of an affected area can be examined under a microscope to confirm the diagnosis. Ringworm is curable but takes weeks to months of treatment, sometimes longer. Recurrence is common and a chronic infection may occur.

Ringworm can occur anywhere on the body. On the skin, ringworm starts as slightly raised, red to brown round patches that itch. As the patch enlarges a central clear area develops – this is where it gets the name "ringworm". Small blisters can occur with ringworm of the groin or feet. Itching is common and can be severe. Scratching can cause bacterial infections in addition to spreading the fungal infection.

Tinea is categorized by where it occurs:

- ♦ Tinea capitis: fungal infection of the scalp (This requires treatment with prescription medications; over-the-counter creams will usually not cure tinea capitis.)
- ♦ Tinea corporis: fungal infection of the body
- ♦ Tinea cruris: fungal infection of the groin (jock itch)
- ♦ Tinea pedis: fungal infection of the feet (athlete's foot)

Wrestlers cannot wrestle in practice or competition with ringworm or tinea.

Treatment

Mild cases of ringworm and tinea can be treated with over-the-counter medications. Use them exactly as directed on the product's label. Read the entire instructions, including the warnings and side effects of any medicines used. Apply a small amount of antifungal cream or ointment (like Lamisil® or Lotrimin®) to affected areas. For athlete's feet, also use a powder (like Desenex®) in all your pairs of shoes. Taking an over-the-counter tablet of Benadryl® (diphenhydramine) by mouth every four to six hours or using an Aveeno® oatmeal bath can help with itching. Hydrocortisone cream (like Cortaid®) can help with itching, redness and irritation. If ringworm is not responsive to over-the-counter medicines, your doctor may recommend a prescription cream to apply to the skin. Continue to use this for 10 days after the infection appears to be completely cured and keep it from coming back. In severe cases that do not respond to medicine applied to the skin, your doctor may give you a prescription medicine taken by mouth. Ringworm of the scalp usually requires weeks to months of treatment with a medication taken by mouth.

DO:

- See your doctor to make the diagnosis, get treatment, and obtain medical clearance.
- Shower and shampoo daily. Gently wash affected areas with a cloth, dry off well (especially your feet), then apply any presecribed creams or ointments to affeted areas. Use your own soap and shampoo.
- Keep moisture away from skin. It is important to keep areas infected with ringworm clean and dry. Always wear clean, dry clothing. Cotton or other absorbent clothing is best. Avoid tight shoes or clothing (like nylon) that chafes your skin.
- Carefully launder all clothing and towels. Change bedding every two days.
- Keep hair cut short and nails trimmed.
- Treat the infection as directed – this will make it heal the quickest. If prescribed topical antifungal creams use them as directed for three to four weeks. If prescribed medication taken by mouth, take them as directed by your doctor. If taking medication by mouth, your doctor may ask you to take a blood test.
- Pets and rodents are a common source of re-infection. Get treatment for pets with skin infections.

DON'T:

- Don't wrestle or workout in the wrestling room until 1) at least five full days of treatment have passed, 2) the area looks completely normal and healed, and 3) you are cleared by your trainer or physician.
- Don't share personal items like headgear, wrestling shoes, razors, combs, brushes, hats, soaps, towels, clothing or bedding.
- Don't scratch.

Never use bleach, peroxide, iodine or other chemical disinfectants. These may not cure it, may scar and may irritate the skin. This may make it look worse to the referee or doctor and delay your return to competition.

CALL YOUR DOCTOR IF:

- If the rash has not improved after two weeks of treatment.
- If signs of a bacterial infection develop such as fever, pus drainage, oozing, crusting, swelling or pain.
- If skin changes occur such as scarring or bleeding.
- If a family member has signs of ringworm.
- Any new, unexpected symptoms or problems occur as some treatments may cause side effects.

For More Information: American Academy of Dermatology, www.aad.org

From *"Championship Nutrition and Performance: The Wrestler's Guide to Lifestyle, Diet and Healthy Weight Control"* by N. Rizzo, M.D., available at **www.wrestlerdiet.com**.

WRESTLING HANDOUT #11: Rules of the Room

Academics & Conduct

♦ Being a responsible wrestler means that you are a responsible student. If your grades are suffering then you are not achieving your goals as a student-athlete.

♦ The best athletes do not have bad grades, unsportsmanlike conduct, or rude behavior. On and off the mats you represent your sport, school, coaches, teammates, parents and yourself. Respect yourself by respecting others and by achieving your best.

♦ All school rules apply at all times to your conduct and behavior as a wrestler.

Wrestling Room Rules & Equipment

♦ No food, drink, or gum is allowed in the wrestling room (except water bottles).

♦ Street shoes are not allowed in the wrestling room.

♦ Wrestling shoes are to be worn only in the wrestling room and during competition.

♦ Do not trim hair or cut nails in the wrestling room.

♦ No wrestling is allowed by an athlete who has not turned in a completed sports physical form, if required by the program or school.

♦ No injured/ill wrestler should wrestle until cleared in writing by a doctor or trainer.

♦ Wrestling is not allowed unless a coach or instructor is present supervising.

♦ You are responsible for your equipment and for replacement costs of any lost gear.

♦ Locks on lockers are required.

Attire

Clothes in the wrestling room should consist of a T-shirt, socks, athletic shorts, and either a jock strap or close-fitting spandex or lycra shorts like bicycling shorts. T-shirts should be new, unripped, properly fitting and cotton. Athletic shorts should be without pockets to prevent fingers or hands getting caught in them. For male athletes a jock strap or pair of bicycling shorts keeps the genitals close to the body and free from injury. (A cup is designed to protect the genitals from direct, hard blows such as from a baseball — as this type of trauma to such a severe degree is not that common in wrestling, a cup may cause more problems than benefits and should not be worn.) Female wrestlers should wear a sports bra under a T-shirt to prevent skin abrasions ("jogger's nipples") or injury. Female wrestlers should not wear hard hair clips or pins, but instead use soft hair restraints or rubber bands. No wrestling clothes should have buttons, zippers, or hard decorative items on them. Boxer shorts are not allowed. To prevent the spread of infections and skin problems all clothing and towels used during practices or meets must be washed every day.

Headgear

There is no benefit of one type of headgear over another. Most, if not all, states require that headgear be worn during all matches. It should be worn during all practices. The headgear should be adjusted so that no strap or other part of the headgear covers the eyes or blocks vision, and the earpieces should rest directly over the ear. The headgear should be comfortable both at rest and when wrestling. Have your coach check the fit of your headgear. Facemasks that attach to the front of the headgear are used when there is a facial injury or when extra protection for the face is needed like a broken nose, soft tissue facial trauma, lip or teeth injuries, or recent/extensive dental procedures.

Mouth Guards

Soft rubber mouth guards are recommended when the athlete has braces or specific dental problems. This serves two functions – it prevents the inside of the lips of the wrestler from being cut when pressure is applied to the face and also prevents cuts and infections on the opposing wrestler. Hard or rigid mouth guards are not recommended, but may be used. Some states may have rules allowing or not allowing certain types of mouth guards.

Elbow and Kneepads

Neither elbow or kneepads have been shown to reduce injuries or help to an injury heal. Despite this, kneepads are commonly worn by wrestlers with knee pain or injury. Possible reasons for this include the idea that the wrestler may feel more confident with the knee protected and the concept of proprioception – that is the ability of the brain to better sense the position of a limb through increased sensory input (the "feel" of the kneepad). Elbow pads can potentially limit the range of motion or control of the arms, especially when wrestling down on the mat, and are not often used.

Shoes & Socks

Properly fitting wrestling shoes should be worn at all times. Wrestling shoes should be worn only in the wrestling room or on the mats at competition. This will maintain the health of the wrestlers by maintaining the shoes in good condition (fewer injuries) and prevent infection spread from mats. Socks should be clean, heavy cotton socks that will help absorb moisture away from the foot. Socks also extend the life of your shoes. Putting antifungal foot powder in your shoes daily will help prevent athlete's foot and other fungal infections.

Wrestling Room Care

The mats should be mopped with an approved mat cleaner or dilute bleach (one part bleach in nine parts water) daily. Mop heads should be changed frequently. Areas in the wrestling room not covered by mats should be vacuumed or swept and then mopped at least once a week. Inspect mats prior to any activity. Specifically identify any deterioration of the covering or foam material. Ensure the integrity of mats mounted to wall surfaces. Repair or replace as required. Mats sections may move during use. Check for proper fastening (taping) prior to use. While some wrestling programs tend to maintain wrestling rooms hot and humid during workouts, this may promote the growth of bacteria and fungus. Keep some access to outside air to help prevent too much humidity during workouts (this will also protect against heat illness). Also, less humid mats are less likely to contribute to "slip" type injuries. Never have a wrestling room with a heat index of 90 or greater – keep the room at a normal temperature and humidity. One rule of thumb is, if the temperature is less than 90° F, to measure the temperature and humidity, and then add them together. If that sum is greater than 130, consider cooling the room off a bit. Another sign that the room is too hot is when signs of heat illness appear (like fatigue, red skin, fast heart rates, moodiness, increased thirst, lack of concentration, etc.), or performance starts to decline.

From **"Championship Nutrition and Performance: The Wrestler's Guide to Lifestyle, Diet and Healthy Weight Control"** by N. Rizzo, M.D., available at **www.wrestlerdiet.com**.

WRESTLING HANDOUT #12: Skin Care

Preventing skin infections can have a huge impact on a wrestler's and a team's success. Many skin problems can be prevented or kept in check by good hygiene and proper medical care. Protecting skin from breaks, scrapes and cuts where infections may enter is an important step. (Commercial skin protectants designed to prevent skin infections are available, but have not yet been proven to work.) This handout describes how to prevent infections through proper skin care.

Once infections like ringworm, impetigo, bacterial folliculitis and herpes show up, a team can pay the price for the entire season. Most of these infections are spread by skin-to-skin-contact, but some like impetigo and folliculitis can also spread via surfaces like pads and handles on weight machines and other wrestler's gear. Because these infections are contagious, they must be recognized and treated right away, and require completely avoiding skin-to-skin contact with other people until complete healing. Any wrestler with open, weeping, pustular or vesicular lesions on the skin must be kept from practice and competition until an accurate diagnosis has been made, proper treatment has been done for sufficient time, and all the lesions have healed. For the coaches and parents infections mean getting wrestlers to doctor appointents, changing lineups, and making sure any skin clearance paperwork is done properly and stays up-to-date. For wrestlers, infections are a serious interruption of their season and development in the sport, in addition to the impact on their health. Wrestling rules do not allow competition with active, contagious skin problems, bandaged or not. Bandaging will not prevent spread to other wrestlers or teammates because bandages become wet, shift and peel off.

Wrestlers with a skin condition must see a physician for diagnosis, treatment and written medical clearance. A referee may request a doctor's written medial clearance before allowing a wrestler to compete, and some states require that specific skin clearance forms be filled out. Keep in mind that some states require that the original form signed by a medical doctor be presented at the time of weigh-in, and a fax or copy is not acceptable. Your doctor may prescribe medicine to control the infection and speed healing. Tell your coach or parents about skin problems right away – ignoring or hiding it will not make it go away.

Finger and Toenails

A wrestler can be disqualified by the referee for having long nails. This rule is in place to help prevent scratches, eye injuries and infections. So fingernails (and toenails) should be kept clean and trimmed at all times. Each wrestler should have his or her own personal pair of nail clippers. Keep a few sets of fingernail clippers (attached to long strings or other objects to keep them from "walking") in the locker room or wrestling office. Replace the clippers when dull. Have a set of clippers in the training bag at meets to catch the one wrestler who forgets. Do not use fingernail clippers on toenails and do not use toenail clippers on fingernails. Using the wrong clippers will result in rougher cuts and more scratches, possible skin damage and infections, and dull or damage the clippers for the next wrestler. Clean clippers with alcohol once a week or more. Don't chew your nails – it may result in torn skin and infection, and it certainly doesn't add any class to the sport.

Hair

Most states' rules require that hair be trimmed at least one inch above the collar. Bangs should never decrease vision. If you have dry skin or dandruff use a quality moisturizing or dandruff shampoo. Use a more expensive brand name as the cheaper brands of shampoo can be drying and irritating to the skin. If you have a skin infection, be sure to inspect the scalp and hair also.

DO:

- If you show *any* signs of infection or have any question about something on your skin tell your coach, parents, team doctor, or family doctor right away.

- Shower with your own soap and shampoo after *every* practice and meet. Showers should be frequently cleaned. Wear shower clogs or similar footwear.

- Keep your skin dry, nails trimmed, hair cut and face clean-shaven.

- Keep skin scrapes and cuts properly bandaged. Clean minor scrapes with soap and water. Use topical antibacterial ointment like Neosporin® or Bacitracin®.

- If athlete's foot or blisters are a problem do the following: Wear properly fitting shoes and gradually break them in. Air out your shoes between uses. As moisture increases friction between skin and fabric, wear a thin pair of socks under thicker, more absorbent socks. Use an antifungal foot power.

- Do not share personal items like clothing, shoes, razors or towels.

- Wash your clothes and towel after *every* practice and meet.

- Use a skin moisturizer or lotion like Vaseline Intensive Care® daily if you have dry skin.

- Take medicines as directed and *only if given to you by your parents or doctor.*

- Clean headgear with a sanitizer like alcohol.

- Keep the wrestling room clean. See WRESTLING HANDOUT #11: Rules of the Room.

- Have a coach, trainer or team doctor do weekly skin, hair and nail checks for the entire team at a weigh out after practice.

DON'T:

- Don't take any pills, creams, or over-the-counter or prescription medicines without your parents' permission and knowledge.

- Do not cut or trim nails or hair in the wrestling room.

- Don't use peroxide, iodine or bleach. These are "chemical" antiseptics and may do more harm than good. Some of these may scar, irritate your skin and make things look worse to the referee or doctor and delay your return to competition or practice.

From *"Championship Nutrition and Performance: The Wrestler's Guide to Lifestyle, Diet and Healthy Weight Control"* by N. Rizzo, M.D., available at **www.wrestlerdiet.com**.

WRESTLING HANDOUT #13: Sprains & Strains*

Strains and sprains are injuries that differ in severity and in which tissues are affected, but are treated in similar ways. With either injury the area will likely be swollen, you may find it difficult to use, move or bear weight on it, and you will have some dull, aching pain in the injured area until completely healed. A strain involves overstretching or overuse of a muscle, ligament or tendon. You may feel pain, weakness or numbness in the injured area. A sprain is the stretching or tearing (partial or complete) of a muscle, ligament or tendon around a joint and usually occurs when the joint is forced to bend further than normal. The symptoms often include a popping or tearing sensation at the time of injury, swelling, and bruising that develop over the next 24 hours. The most common sprain is the ankle sprain, which is when the foot is turned inward and your full weight comes down on the ankle. A sprain is more serious than a strain and requires more intense treatment. Almost all resolve completely without further problems.

Treatment

Proper treatment will help prevent swelling, protect the joint until it heals, prevent muscle weakness, and get you moving again as quickly as possible. The initial treatment consists of five parts, represented by the term **PRICE**. Remember the term **PRICE** and what it stands for, and you will know how to treat a strain or sprain.

P = Protect. Protect the part from re-injury. While it is good to keep the joint moving, you must avoid a second injury before the first one heals. This may mean not returning to the sport until you are completely healed. Use crutches or splints if you are advised to.

R = Rest. Rest the joint for at least one to two days. Again, the severity of the injury will determine how long you need to rest the limb.

I = Ice. Apply ice immediately because the swelling can start in a few minutes. Continue icing several times a day (15 minutes at a time) for two to three days, or longer depending on how severe your injury is.

C = Compression. Compress the area firmly (but not too tightly) with a stretch-type bandage like an ACE® bandage. Some serious sprains may require a cast, a splint, a brace or an air cast. Whichever bandage or splint is used should be wrapped firmly around the injury, but not so tightly that blood flow is restricted.

E = Elevation. Elevate the injured part to at least heart level as much as possible to help reduce swelling. But don't elevate too high because you could reduce blood flow. For an injured arm, keep the arm in a sling while you are up and about. When lying down, elevate the arm on pillows or across the chest. For an injured hand, try to keep it higher than the elbow. For an injured lower limb, elevate the injured part on pillows or a chair. The foot should be higher than the knee or hip.

The next treatment is protected motion that allows the ankle to move without moving too far and further injuring the joint. This may be as simple as using a compression wrap, splint or brace. After your initial recovery, your doctor may prescribe physical therapy to speed healing and help prevent future injury. Some forms of physical therapy help keep muscles from weakening and help remove any swelling. Other types may improve proprioception (the ability to know the position of your limb without looking at it). Sometimes your doctor may suggest heat, or alternating cold and heat. Severe injuries may require casting or even surgery when the ligaments are completely torn or if there are multiple ligaments injured.

DO:

♦ Take any medicines prescribed by your doctor. Some over-the-counter medications may be used for less severe sprains, but only with your parents' permission.

♦ You should follow the instructions for **PRICE** immediately after your injury.

♦ Do any physical therapy prescribed by your doctor.

♦ Frequently move or stretch the fingers or toes of an immobilized limb to help circulation and decrease swelling.

♦ Compare the injured limb to the other limb. This is a good way to notice warning signs like changes in color, temperature and swelling.

DON'T:

♦ Don't do activities that will increase swelling because this will slow your return to complete activity. Too much activity, standing or sitting with the injured limb hanging down should be avoided.

♦ Don't use heat for the first 72 hours after the injury because it will nearly always cause more swelling that will slow recovery.

♦ Don't use aspirin for the first 48 hours. Tylenol® (acetaminophen) is okay.

♦ Don't wear rings or bracelets on an injured limb.

♦ If your doctor gives you a splint, don't remove or reshape it – talk to your doctor if it is uncomfortable. If wrapping is too tight, loosen it.

CALL YOUR DOCTOR IF:

♦ If swelling is increasing, (the skin around it should not be tight).

♦ If it feels warm or hot. (The injured part is usually cooler than surrounding tissues.)

♦ If you feel a sudden increase in the type or severity of pain.

♦ If the area is very red, purple or blue – this is different from bruised areas that are usually bluish. (The injured part is usually paler than the surrounding flesh.)

♦ If you can't bend your fingers or toes, even though it might hurt a little.

♦ If you keep a shoe on or if your doctor wraps the injured area in a bandage, cast, splint or compression wrap you should watch for signs that it is getting too tight and cutting off the blood supply to the injured area, or the hands, fingers, feet or toes. It can also press on muscles and nerves and damage them. Symptoms in the fingers and toes on the injured limb would include numbness, tingling, feeling as if they are asleep, blueness, duskiness or coldness. If any of these occur, check the circulation (pulse), loosen whatever is tight and call your doctor.

♦ You are not noticing significant improvement within seven to ten days.

♦ There is any popping, catching or giving way of the joint after the swelling has gone away. These may be signs of a more severe injury than was originally thought.

*Refer also to WRESTLING HANDOUT #14: When to Use Heat and Cold for Injuries.

From *"Championship Nutrition and Performance: The Wrestler's Guide to Lifestyle, Diet and Healthy Weight Control"* by N. Rizzo, M.D., available at **www.wrestlerdiet.com**.

WRESTLING HANDOUT #14: When to Use Heat & Cold for Athletic Injuries

Common injuries seen in athletics are bruises (contusions), muscle pulls (strains), sprains and fractures. A contusion is a bruise without a break in the skin, usually caused by a hard blow to a muscle. The result is internal bleeding, swelling, and pain with movement. Muscle pulls or strains occur when muscle or tendon is damaged by a contraction while it is under excessive strain. The muscle fibers stretch and tear, resulting in internal bleeding and swelling. Strains usually involve the quadriceps, hamstrings and calf muscles. A sprain is an injury to the ligament of a joint. Sprains occur when a joint is forced beyond its normal range of motion. Swelling is usually great and the pain can be severe. An important question is whether to use heat or cold in treating the injury. A general guideline to follow is to use cold in the early stage of most injuries then use heat later for certain types of injuries. Remember "**PRICE**" as a guide to treating acute injuries. **PRICE** stands for **Protect** the injured part from further injury; **Rest** the injury; apply **Ice**; apply **Compression** firmly (but not too tightly); and **Elevate** the injury to decrease bleeding.

How Cold Works

Using cold with gentle compression after you suffer an injury helps stop internal bleeding in the tissue, relieve pain, reduce muscle spasms, cool deep tissues, lower metabolic activity, and reduce swelling and inflammation. It can produce dramatic drops in tissue swelling because cold initially constricts the walls of blood vessels and decreases blood flow to the injured tissue. Compression also decreases the blood flow to an injured body part. *If you feel pain with gentle compression contact your physician immediately.* (Also, elevation, helps to "drain" excess fluid from injured areas.) Compared to heat, cold works better to decrease swelling and discomfort.

Cold's pain-killing effect is caused by its "deadening" of nerve activity; patients who use cold therapy on injuries tend to require much less pain medication. It also creates a "window of pain relief" during rehabilitation so that patients can reestablish normal motion. This effect, though, can sometimes be counterproductive; an athlete who has iced down an injured body part may get so much pain relief that he/she returns to activity too soon. Cold decreases muscle spasms by making muscles less sensitive to being stretched, and, like heat, cold can be used to treat low-back pain. (As an aside, research suggests that cold works better for individuals who have had back pain for more than 14 days, while heat may be more effective for those with more recent pain.)

When to Use Cold

Cold therapy is used for contusions, muscle pulls and strains, sprains and fractures. *PRICE* is the recommended treatment. Apply ice with pressure and elevate the limb. Activity can be resumed gradually after the pain and swelling have gone and full use of the limb has returned. Cold eases pain and helps restore motion.

How to Apply Cold Therapy

The earlier the cold is started the better. You should apply ice as soon as possible after the injury and continue using it for the next two or three days, or until the swelling goes away. Don't place ice or ice packs directly on the injury site – you could suffer frostbite. Place the ice pack over a wet towel or washcloth and use an elastic bandage to hold the ice pack in place. Apply the ice pack to the injury site for ten to 15 minutes every three to four hours while awake. However, individuals with large amounts of fat under their skin may require longer periods of icing (but no longer than 20 minutes). An ice massage is a good way to treat an overuse injury. Freeze water in a paper or styrofoam cup. Then tear away the cup's top lip and rub the ice over the injured area for five to ten minutes. If you are unable to tolerate cold therapy, do not use it.

Apply cold therapy daily until the discoloration and swelling are gone. Exercises to regain full use of the injured area should be started as soon as possible. It is important to allow some mobility during icing. Instead of sitting around with ice packs on, try taking a roll of plastic wrap, cut it down the middle, and use the half roll as a quick "sports wrap" to easily and firmly secure the ice pack over a treatment area. This makes it easier for you to follow through with your icing properly.

Ice chips in a plastic bag are most effective, followed by the use of frozen gel packs and blue ice packs, which are better than chemical reaction packs or gas refrigerant-filled packs.

How Heat Works
The application of superficial heat to your body can improve the flexibility of your tendons and ligaments, reduce muscle spasms, alleviate pain, elevate blood flow and boost metabolism. Exactly how heat relieves pain is not exactly known, although some believe that it inactivates nerve fibers which can force muscles into irritating spasms, and that it may cause the release of endorphins (powerful body chemicals which block pain transmission). Heat does help tissue rebuild by increasing blood flow and tissue repair. Increased blood flow occurs in heated parts of the body because heat tends to relax the walls of blood vessels. That's why sports doctors recommend that you do not heat up already inflamed joints.

When to Use Heat
Heat therapy can be used during the repair stage of an injury when new tissue is being formed. This is usually 48 to 72 hours after the initial injury (once the risk of internal bleeding is minimal), and after ice has been used and swelling is reduced. That's because heat increases the blood flow to the injury area, and that can increase swelling. Heat in any form should not be applied to an acute injury or where discoloration or swelling is present.

While heat shouldn't be used to treat an acute injury, it can be used to reduce muscle spasms, increase flexibility, decrease joint stiffness and limber up soft tissue. It can loosen tight muscles and joints during a warm-up before you exercise, possibly preventing injury. Moist heat is good for muscles that are sore, tired or overworked. Heat and massage also help shinsplints. Heat is effective for treatment of muscle cramps along with stretching and massage. Although heat can reduce muscle spasms after a back injury (which is usually muscular), heat should not be used on ligament injuries like sprained ankles or strained joints. Heat should not be applied to infants or elderly persons.

How to Apply Heat Therapy
Hot water bottles, heating pads on the lowest setting, warm soaks in the tub or shower, and warm moist towels are effective sources of heat. The heat should not come in direct contact with the skin. Apply heat for 15 to 20 minutes at a time. The proper tissue temperature for heating is probably 104° to 113° Fahrenheit (40° to 45° Celsius) and the correct application time is about five to 30 minutes. Apply heat for three to four days and begin stretching exercises. Do not sleep on your heat source. Always check the temperature of the heat source to prevent accidental burns.

* Refer also to WRESTLING HANDOUT #13: Sprains and Strains.

From *"Championship Nutrition and Performance: The Wrestler's Guide to Lifestyle, Diet and Healthy Weight Control"* by N. Rizzo, M.D., available at **www.wrestlerdiet.com**.

REFERENCES

1. Landry, R., Oppliger, R., Shelter, A., & Landry, G., The Wrestler's Diet: A Guide to Healthy Weight Control, Chicago: Quaker Oats Company, 1991.

2. Perriello, V., Aiming for Healthy Weight in Wrestlers and Other Athletes. *Contemporary Pediatrics* 18(9): 55-74. September 2001.

3. Roberts, W., Certifying Wrestlers' Minimum Weight: A New Requirement. *The Physician and Sports Medicine,* 26(10). Minneapolis: McGraw- Hill, October 1998.

4. Oppliger, Case, Horswill, Landry and Shelter. American College of Sports Medicine. Position Stand: Weight Loss in Wrestlers. *Medicine & Science in Sports & Exercise* 28(6): 9-12, June 1996.

5. Eichner, E.R., Muscle Cramps: The Right Ways for the Dog Days, Gatorade Sports Science Institute, copyright 2002, URL: http://www.gssi.com.

6. Clark, N., Eating Before Competing, *The Physician and Sports Medicine*, 26(9), Minneapolis: McGraw- Hill, 1998.

7. Oppliger, Harms, Herrmann, Streich and Clark. The Wisconsin Wrestling Minimum Weight Project: a Model for Weight Control Among High School Wrestlers. *Medicine & Science in Sports & Exercise* 27(8): 1220-1224, August 1995.

8. Anderson, S., A.T.C., Hellickson, M.A., Landry, G., M.D., Sossin, K, M.S., C.D.N.: Sports Science Exchange Roundtable: Training and Nutrition For Amateur Wrestling, Gatorade Sports Science Institute, copyright 2000 URL: http://www.gssi.com.

9. Mysnyk, M.C., Snook, G.A., Sports Injuries: Mechanisms, Prevention, and Treatment, edited by Fu, F., Stone, D., Wrestling: (43): 715-727, New York: Lippincot Williams and Wilkins, 1994.

10. Dalen, K., R.N., M.S.N., C.F.N.P., Giddens, J., R.N., M.S.N., C.S., Miller, D., R.N., B.S.N., Mitchell, P., R.N., M.S.N., Thompson, J., R.N., Dr. P.H., Tucker, S., R.N., M.S.N., P.H.N., C.N.A.A., Mosby-Year Book, Patient Teaching Guides, Update III. p. 240. St. Louis: Mosby, 1998.

11. Tackett, C., Understanding Labels and Health Claims – Part One. Global Health & Fitness, copyright 1997 - 2003, URL: http://www.global-fitness.com.

12. Casa, D., Ph.D., A.T.C., C.S.C.S.; Armstrong, L., Ph.D., F.A.C.S.M., Hillman, S., M.S., M.A., A.T.C., P.T., Montain, S., Ph.D., F.A.C.S.M.; Reiff, R., M.Ed., A.T.C.; Rich, B., M.D., ATC; William O. Roberts, MD, F.A.C.S.M.; Stone, J., M.S., A.T.C.: National Athletic Trainers' Association Position Statement: Fluid Replacement for Athletes, *Journal of Athletic Training:* 35(2): 212-224.

13. Benardot, D., Ph.D., Nutrition for Serious Athletes. Champaign: Human Kinetics, 2000.

14. Vickery, D., M.D., Fries, J., M.D., Take Care of Yourself. Cambridge: Perseus Books, 2001.

15. The National Eating Disorder Information Center, copyright, 2003, URL: http://www.nedic.com.

16. Karpay, E., The Everything Total Fitness Book, Avon: Adams Media Corporation, 2000.

17. Neporent, L., Scholsberg, S., Weight Training For Dummies, 2nd ed., New York: Hungry Minds, Inc., 2000.

18. Casey, J. M.D., Is There a Magic Weight Loss Carb?, copyright 2003, URL: http://www.webmd.com.

19. Skinner, R., R.D., M.S., L.D., CSCS, Nutrition for Muscle Mass, Gatorade Sports Science Institute, copyright 2002, URL: http://www.gssi.com.

20. Sandor, R., M.D., Heat Illness, *The Physician and Sports Medicine*, 25(6). Minneapolis: McGraw- Hill, 1997.

21. Cantor, M. Ph.D.: Coaches' Corner, Refueling for Stop-and-Go Sports, Gatorade Sports Science Institute, copyright 1996, URL: http://www.gssi.com.

22. Sarnataro, B., Whole Foods Best for Workouts: Only Elite Athletes Need Supplements and Energy Bars. The Rest of Us Can Fuel Our Workouts With Regular Whole Foods., copyright 2003, URL: http://www.webmd.com.

23. National Institue of Diabetes and Digestive and Kidney Diseases, Weight-Control Information Network, Just Enough For You: About Food Portions, copyright 2003, URL: http://www.niddk.nih.gov/health/nutrit/nutrit.htm.

24. Mann, D., WebMD Feature Archive, Buyer Beware: Energy Bars May Be No Better Than Bagels, copyright 2002, URL: http://webmd.com.

25. Food Guide Pyramid: Guide to Daily Food Choices, US Department of Agriculture, US Department of Health and Human Services, as cited by Nelson, J., Mayo Clinic Diet Manual: a Handbook of Nutrition Practices, Chicago: Mosby, 1994.

26. Gatorade Sports Science Institute, Exchange Roundtable: Training Youth in Sport: Nutritional Needs, Roundtable #30/Vol. 8, No. 4, copyright 1997, URL: http://www.gssi.com.

27. The Truth About Carbs: Their Role in Healthy, Long-Term Weight Loss, New York: WeightWatchers International, Inc., copyright 2003.

28. Willett, Walter, C., M.D., Eat, Drink, and Be Healthy, New York: Simon & Schuster, 2001.

29. Parker-Pope, T., How to Give Your Child A Longer Life, The Wall Street Journal Online on AOL, copyright 2003, URL: http://www.aol.com.

30. The Center for Nutrition in Sport and Human Performance, Taking it to the Mat: The Wrestler's Guide for Optimal Performance, Amherst: Univeristy of Massachusetts, copyright 2003.

Nicholas Rizzo, M.D.

INDEX

NOTES

NOTES

AUTHOR RECOMMENDATION: A key part of training is knowing what you have done, where you are now, and where you need to be. To help accomplish this, use

"The ARSENAL: The Wrestler's Training Log"
By NCAA National Champion Alan Fried, Oklahoma State University
available at www.wrestlerdiet.com or www.arsenaltraining.com.

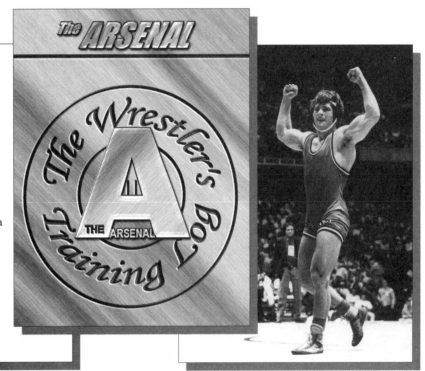

"One does not become a champion by accident! Being a champion requires constant planning and analysis of your performance. This training log will help you create your road map to success."

– Kendall Cross, 1996
   Olympic Champion, 1990
   NCAA Champion

"To reach your goals you need a plan. You can't do it randomly. You must train, then compete, then evaluate and do that process over and over again. This training log puts all of this and more at your fingertips."

– Bruce Burnett, USA
   Olympic Head Coach

- 52-week journal formatted specifically for all options in a wrestler's training day
- Three workouts broken down into: Strength / Conditioning / Technique / Wrestling
- Daily entry of a.m. & p.m. body weight for proper weight control
- Weekly attention to: Injury rehab / Scouting / Total training hours / Goal progress
- Chapters on "Care of Strains & Sprains" and "When to Use Heat & Cold for Athletic Injuries" from *"Championship Nutrition and Performance"* by Nicholas Rizzo, M.D.
- Complete weight training program
- Detailed match and tournament result entry
- Strength and conditioning performance tests
- Effective advice on goal setting
- Activity specific calorie burning reference chart
- 1000-food detailed calorie counter

Alan Fried is a rare three-time NCAA finalist, claiming the top spot in 1994 and finishing with a career collegiate record of 129-6. He also owns two University and two Espoir (20 yrs. and under) National Freestyle Championships and became the Espoir World Freestyle Champion in 1991, where he was voted Best Technical Wrestler of the tournament.

Alan Fried earned his B.S. in Psychology from Oklahoma State University in 1994 and his Juris Doctorate from The Cleveland-Marshall College of Law in 2002, winning both the CALI Excellence for the Future and Charles Auerbach Memorial Awards for outstanding achievement.